WHAT THE`

"High praises for the book postpartum is forever!!!! This book is a practical and comprehensive guide for women throughout the lifespan. I love it that Jessica begins with educating women from A younger age….. finally!! Self-care in a woman's 20s can be a game changer in optimizing health during pregnancy and postpartum but also in preventing problems during that time and throughout menopause. Knowledge is power and Jessica does an amazing job of empowering women in this book. I hope all women and practitioners read this book to improve self awareness and self care. Jessica sets the stage of creating the level of Pelvic Health that all women deserve!"

—Susan Winograd, MSPT,
owner of Pelvicore Rehab
www.pelvicorerehab.com

"Dr. Papa delivers an honest and introspective look at the process of conception, pregnancy, and post-partum periods in a woman's life. This book provides easy to comprehend overviews of what to expect and how to manage common issues that many women face during these precious yet sometimes challenging periods of life. With bravery she discusses her own experiences and provides clinical perspectives to help ease any struggles."

—Dr. Amanda Olson, DPT, PRPC
Intimate Rose
Www.IntimateRose.com

"This book will never go out of style! Dr. Jessica Papa has written a bible for women's health. Here is a touchy subject for most people, but she brilliantly explains what is going on in our bodies without causing any embarrassing moments. Dr. Papa takes us from youth to maturity helping us understand what goes on inside and how to take steps to help. Most women feel their reproductive parts have no say in healing. Not according to Dr. Papa, she discusses the hows and whys and then offers natural solutions. The moment I picked up this book I wanted to read it from cover to cover. Thank-you, Dr. Papa for helping ALL women understand what goes on in the the pelvic floor and giving us hope and knowledge for healing and health."

—Dorothy McGuinness, PT
Author of "SIMPLE HEALING, 5 Steps to Heal the Body and Soul"

"This book is such a wealth of information for women preparing for pregnancy and who are in the postpartum phase of life. It is a wonderful guide in all the ways we can help ourselves have a more positive experience all around. This book simplifies the postpartum phase in order to easily and practically guide you back to feeling strong and confident again. Highly recommend this book to anyone who is pregnant or postpartum."

—Dr. Nicole Laird, PT, DPT
Owner of Hays County PT
www.hayscountypt.com

Weaving together her extensive knowledge of the human body, her own personal journey and years of research Dr. Jess beautifully pulls back the veil on the postpartum experience in her latest book Postpartum is Forever. Many birthing people dedicate much of their pregnancy to preparing for their labor and birth, while downplaying the importance of learning about how their unique path will directly impact their life moving forward. It is essential that we take an active role in our wellness. As a doula, I will absolutely be encouraging my clients and friends to add this to their "must-read" lists!

—Barbie French, CD(DONA)
www.naturesom.com

POST**PARTUM**
IS
FOREVER

A Pelvic Health Specialist's Guide to
Heal and Optimize Your Body **Before**,
During *and* **After** Pregnancy

Dr. Jessica L. Papa

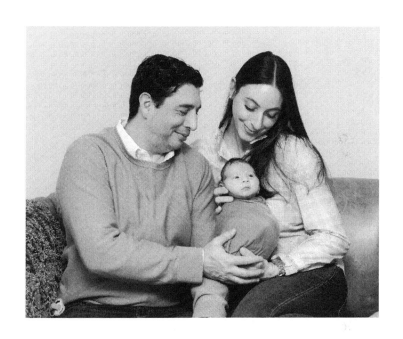

*To my husband, Steven for your patience, love,
friendship, and willingness to eat takeout.*

*And also to my son, Theodore
You are so loved, for the boy you are, the man you will
become and the precious son you will always be.*

Hey Mama,

The journey to physical therapy is a personal one. No matter the reason you found yourself here, know that you are taking the right steps. As a Myofascial Release Expert, I specialize in helping women navigate health concerns surrounding trauma, pregnancy, chronic pain, and bladder issues. When it comes to these female-specific problems, I know that your voice may have been drowned out or even silenced. That, my friend, is never okay. Today, you will learn that you are not alone and that pain and discomfort should never have a stronghold over any stage of womanhood.

This is your guide from puberty, through pregnancy, and into your twilight years. Everything you need to know about how to care for your body in this stage, what to expect in the next, and preventative care in the now is right here in your hands. Your voice is strong and loud, let us speak up together and take back our power when it comes to pelvic health.

This book will provide you with valuable information to start feeling better right away! I want to provide you with the best information possible to get you on the road toward resuming all of what you want to do in life. While I cannot promise you that these tips will work for every single person, every single time, it is certainly better than spending another day putting up with pain, avoiding activities that you love, or relying on pain medication.

It doesn't matter whether you're quite young, are raising your kids, have no kids, or have kids that are long since out of the house. It doesn't matter whether you are a high-level athlete or whether you get very little routine exercise. What does matter is that you have the most up-to-date and accurate information so that you can begin thinking about your pelvic health before you become pregnant or before you start displaying signs and symptoms of pelvic dysfunction. Through targeted work, we have the power to prevent, or greatly minimize, potential pelvic issues and encourage faster, smoother recovery from pelvic dysfunction, surgeries, and childbirth.

Treat your body with kindness wherever you find yourself.

With love,
Dr. Jess

CONTENTS

BEGIN WITH HOPE

I was destined to be a mother. I felt that deep, deep down. It was a part of me that had been there before I could recognize what it was and something that guided my decisions, my relationships, and my fears. I was a mother in the making.

I had always thought of myself as a younger mom; my plan was to be married and expecting in my mid-20s. Life did not exactly go to plan, of course, as it tends to do. This was an issue. I am what you would call type A. I like to plan. I like for my plans to have plans. In fact, if I could, I would have plans A-Z ready for every conceivable moment of my life. An early marriage to the wrong man, losing loved ones before I was ready, and changes in my career all taught me that those plans I made and would make were merely suggestions.

Eventually, life brought me to the place I was meant to be and I met the love of my life. When Steven and I were married in 2020, we waited almost a full year before we started to try for that sweet baby that had been taking up space in my head and heart for so long. I knew the risks associated with my age, now that I was about a decade older than I originally hoped, and I was determined to be proactive in my reproduction. I did what I do best and prepared and I read the books, ate healthy, all of that good stuff. When I was ready to get serious I went to a local acupuncturist who specializes in fertility. After three weeks of treatment and four months of actively trying, I got it—a positive pregnancy test.

I found out when I was only four weeks pregnant, meaning that I got my first positive home pregnancy test a full ten weeks before most women. Those first few weeks were like a dream. I took at least a dozen over-the-counter tests to confirm before ringing up my doctor and scheduling a blood draw to make it official. That confirmation brought so much joy to us and we started bonding with the little life growing.

My fifth week of pregnancy was the end of that dream. It began in the mornings. Between waking up in the morning and lunch, I was feeling…off. I was fatigued to the point of falling asleep in the middle of the day, and experiencing symptoms I had not planned for. I figured it was just a natural part of pregnancy, something that my doctor confirmed as well. The day before what would mark my sixth week, I took a deep, heavy nap in the afternoon. When I woke up, I went to use the restroom.

The instant I saw the blood in the bowl, I knew. I was experiencing a miscarriage before I had even had my first OB visit and work-up. The sight of the blood made me burst into uncontrollable tears. This lasted all night and into the next morning. I woke up feeling a heaviness in my heart. I had lost my baby and, at the time, I thought, also my hope.

I did not know then, what I know now: that hope cannot be lost, not truly. It can only seem small and far away. If you call it with love, it will always find its way home.

THE MANY STAGES OF
A WOMAN'S BODY

Sometimes it feels like I am giving the inevitable truth that I am always aging a big middle finger when I'm slathering on my anti-wrinkle moisturizer or plucking a stray gray hair from the crown of my head. Other times, I feel like I am giving it a big hug as I climb into bed at 8:00 p.m. for an early night of reading with my husband. I know it is there in the tick of the clock and in the hazy memories of my earlier days, waiting and watching. It took me longer than I would like to admit to recognizing that though the waning of time is a constant companion, it is not the villain in my story.

The world tries to tell us that holding on to the state our body was in as a young adult is the pinnacle of beauty and health. I say that the definition of beauty and health will change with you. Understanding the various changes your body goes through as you grow older is essential in keeping your body in its best shape possible to promote a healthier life. Embracing it is the key to continued health and happiness.

Each change represents a new stage and each new stage comes with its own unique benefits and challenges. Navigating these stages of womanhood means meeting those painful, scary, and wonderful moments with grace. By anticipating when changes will come and welcoming the new stage we are entering, we can once again retain the autonomy that we deserve.

For the purpose of this book, we will classify each stage of womanhood by the standard hormonal changes we can all expect. This would be infancy, puberty, reproductive age, climacteric period, and elderly years. We will not only prepare ourselves for the upcoming changes in our life, but also learn to celebrate them.

The Reproductive Years

The 20s - The Beginning

This stage encompasses late teens to women who are yet to reach menopause. It is when most of us feel our "best." Our bodies in our 20s produce the female hormones estrogen, androgen, and progesterone at peak levels, thus promoting more fats and muscles than our adolescent years. At this stage, we tend to begin to have a more consistent menstrual flow due to a more regular ovulation cycle. This is also when many women first experience tender breasts, cramps, and premenstrual syndrome (PMS).

While women in this group are generally healthy and lively, they should exercise and eat well to avoid diseases like diabetes and other chronic diseases. It would help if you also underwent routine medical checks for breast cancer, skin cancer (melanoma), elevated cholesterol, and blood pressure to prevent future complications associated with aging and hormonal changes.

The 30s - Unexplored Changes

Women in their 30s and older also go through physical changes. Though this is also a fertile period, you are most likely of any demographic to experience miscarriage and other pregnancy-related issues. Some may even have problems with maintaining a healthy weight, reducing stress, and maintaining youthful skin. This is due to the intense hormonal changes that are bound to occur as your body changes to accommodate each new phase of life.

However, we can reduce the chances of facing these issues by maintaining a healthier lifestyle. It is important to avoid smoking and the abuse of both prescription and illegal drugs. Also, wear sunscreen to protect your skin against the ultraviolet rays' impact and frequently monitor your body mass index (BMI), cholesterol, and blood pressure.

Your 30s can be a time of renewal for many women. We are often entering motherhood or finally getting into the groove of it. Some of us are finding success in our careers and allocating time to our exercise and diets. Our bodies are different from when we were 20, but not worse or better.

The 40s - Bigger Changes

We should be on the lookout for stress in our 40s. Stress has been shown to lead to depression, high blood pressure, insomnia, and heart diseases—all issues that become prevalent for this age group. These years may also come with bone density mineral loss, as seen in studies[1] that indicate that as we advance in age, so does the incidence of osteopenia and osteoporosis.[2] We may want to counteract it with routine fitness exercises that build muscle and make you stronger. Exercise also keeps your weight in check, reduces your risk of developing cancer, depression, and other unpleasant symptoms of menopause.

While generally menopause is expected when a woman reaches her late 40s, some women become menopausal earlier or later than expected. Women are quite strong and active at this reproductive stage, yet physiological changes within the body might lead to ovarian or uterine diseases and menstrual disorders. We might experience increased bone loss (can be counteracted by calcium intake), premenstrual syndrome, dysmenorrhea, night sweats, sleepless nights, and heart palpitation.

Fortunately, a healthy lifestyle can prevent or lessen the undesirable effects of most of these changes. Your physician can be your best friend as you navigate these years. Never be afraid to reach out and ask questions. Your body is valuable and respecting it as such is a beautiful thing.

Pregnancy

During the childbearing years, we are statistically likely to experience pregnancy. Pregnancy begins the moment the developing embryo implants in the womb. Some women experience minimal bleeding when this occurs; however, others do not have this experience. After implantation, the placenta forms, and the umbilical cord connects the fetus and mother at the placenta to exchange food nutrients, eliminate waste, and exchange gas.

The common signs of pregnancy include a missed menstrual period, breast tenderness, increased basal body temperature, darkening of the cervix, vulva, and the vagina, among many other symptoms. As women, most of us are experienced in identifying some of these symptoms. Others, not so much.

Healthcare workers also look out for other hormonal and physical changes during pregnancy tests. These changes typically happen within the first 12 weeks, known as the first trimester. During this time, pregnant women may experience some morning sickness.

The second trimester occurs from the 13th to the 28th week. During this phase, most women gain weight, and they feel better as the morning sickness gradually fades away. By the end of the 28th week, people can easily see a woman's protruding tummy. The womb expands 20 times its size, and the fetus's movement, known as quickening, starts being felt at this stage of the pregnancy.

The third and final trimester is between weeks 29 to 40. Expectant mothers gain more weight, their abdomen drops, the pelvis tilts, and the back arches to help keep balance. The abdominal muscles stretch, producing a poor posture, causing a change in walking style.

During gestation, the phase between conception and birth, the breakdown and absorption of food changes within the expectant mother to provide the growing fetus enough nutrients for adequate development. These hormonal changes can cause cravings and an increased appetite for food. Fluid retention adds to the increasing body weight to increase the length and width of the foot. The increased production of hormones, like estrogen and relaxin, during pregnancy, causes certain skeletal joints to increase in laxity and widen.

Physicians recommend moderate exercise during pregnancy to improve physical fitness and improve the general circulation of gasses and nutrients. This recommendation is necessary as care needs to be taken to accommodate the various hormonal and metabolic changes during pregnancy.

Pregnancy can be seen as one of, if not, the biggest life event we may experience. For many, it serves as a divider in our health and many long-term health issues can be traced back to this stage. Once we have experienced pregnancy, we will forevermore be postpartum. Embracing this allows us to find beauty in the new way that our bodies work.

Remember this: "Just do your Kegels" is fake news! Kegels are not preparing your pelvic floor for childbirth. No matter what your pregnancy app, birth class, OBGYN, or that pregnant influencer tells you, Kegels are not the answer. In fact, Kegels can do more harm than good as we prepare our pelvic floor for birth.

Postpartum

Postpartum begins right after we give birth, and it is associated with specific changes in the body you must not overlook. For instance, some women feel the urge to urinate more frequently because pregnancy puts pressure on the pelvic muscles. However, it is common for women to release some urine when they sneeze, laugh, or exercise even after birth. All these are symptoms of issues with the pelvic floor due to childbirth, known as **stress incontinence.**

If you experience such symptoms, you might want to consider making some healthy lifestyle changes, or you could report to your doctor for help. Reaching out to medical professionals should be a first resort, not the last. Stress incontinence is common, but should not be considered as normal and it should be treated under the care of someone who understands your body from the inside out. Consider researching PTs in your area that specialize in women's health. This will be your most utilized resource as you begin to treat your body because your PT will know exactly how to assess your current health and can plan your treatment in accordance with your needs and lifestyle.

I am aware of the difficulties in putting this into practice. The fear of embarrassment, the many hoops insurance companies ask you to jump through, even the accessibility to local clinics can stand in the way of proper treatment. Together, we can find a way around it all. You should know that most states now have direct access, which means you don't need a doctor's referral to begin seeing a therapist. It is within your rights to reach out to any medical professional that you believe can help you, without going through a third party.

Some look outside of official medical advice when it comes to stress incontinence as well. If you have already gone down the rabbit hole that is your Google search engine, you have probably seen the countless articles and blog posts that tout the benefits of Kegeling. Unfortunately, this popular exercise of the pelvic floor is not usually the answer and can actually contribute to worsening symptoms in the long run. All pelvic floor exercises should be performed under the guidance of pelvic health physical therapists.

After childbirth, some women also feel pain during sex. These circumstances occur because breastfeeding suppresses the production of estrogen, which lubricates the vagina during sex. The first precaution is to engage only in slow sex, after which you resort to an obstetrician/gynecologist if the pain persists. Doctors often recommend an over-the-counter lubrication product. A second possible cause of this pain is pelvic floor dysfunction or a tear during vaginal birth. Women who have undergone a C-section, on the other hand, also feel pain during sex because both C-sections and pregnancy tighten or stretch muscles.

A handful of women also experience pelvic organ prolapse, a situation where an organ that has shifted from its original position presses against the vaginal wall, causing a feeling of pressure in the vagina.

If the pressure is mild, it can be alleviated by lying down. Also, exhale when lifting heavy objects and do not bear down when pooping. This condition can be fixed using support in the vagina to push up the organ or be corrected through surgery. However, it is best to see your doctor for treatment.

Another postpartum condition that often goes overlooked is diastasis recti. This is a separation of the abdominal muscles as a result of excessive stretching of the abdomen. If a woman has a difficult time returning her abdominals back to their original state, she may have experienced diastasis recti. This condition can be repaired with exercises, and in extreme cases, surgery. Women should assess themselves to see if this condition affects them. If so, then seek professional help.

Postpartum, a woman has to take care of her muscles. It would help if you carry your baby on both sides and sit up properly to avoid much stress on your muscles. But in most medical situations, it's advisable to talk to your physical therapist for help. Postpartum symptoms that are serious and require immediate medical attention include:

- Seizures
- Pain in the chest
- A cut that is not healing
- Shortness of breath
- Persistent headache
- Reduced vision quality

While postpartum is forever and incontinence is common, it should not be taken lightly or perceived to be usual. Physical therapy (prehab) before delivery is so important. It can drastically reduce the chances and severity of pelvic pressure, which causes incontinence and other issues like pain with sitting, low back pain, pain during intercourse, and other complications. Also, talk to your physician if you're faced with any pregnancy-related disease, such as high blood pressure or gestational diabetes.

This is also the time that you may feel the most pressure to wear your body out, attempting to retain the stage of life you were in before pregnancy, an impossible standard. We will explore the many ways that you can take care of the new you by allowing yourself to experience this stage without the guilt and without the fear.

The Climacteric Period

The climacteric period represents the five years before and after menopause. The most common sign of perimenopause is a change in your menstrual cycle. Generally, a woman can be at the menopause stage if she experiences no menstruation for 12 consecutive months. This occurrence is typical in women from 45 through 55 years old. There is a decrease in estrogen levels at this age range, resulting in vasomotor symptoms like vertigo, thinner and dryer skin, excessive sweating, hot flushes, inconsistent urinating, migraines, and the common mood changes we all know to be associated with menopause. These symptoms may be experienced at different levels by different women, although some lucky women do not have any of these symptoms.

Medical conditions such as osteoporosis, hypercholesterolemia, and atherosclerosis may arise due to hormonal changes. However, these diseases are also affected by lifestyle and could be avoided by women with very healthy lifestyles. Women who experience severe symptoms should see their physicians for help. At this stage, it's advisable to regularly screen for breast and uterine cancer, blood pressure, cholesterol, density tests for osteoporosis, neurological diseases, and skin screening as the worst conditions can be avoided by early detection.

Our society has a bad habit of treating bodies at this stage like a car on its last leg. We see less representation in the media and the changes that we are expected to undergo are discussed only in private or under the guise of a joke. Let's lift the mask off of this stage and allow ourselves to see the beauty in it.

Post-climacteric (elderly) Years

Women experience very little to no ovarian function during the post-climactic stage. The elderly experience a decline in physical strength and loss of memory. People in this group should make conscious efforts to regularly visit their physician to avoid high-risk diseases, such as dementia, cerebral and cardiac diseases, and malignant neoplasm.

A woman's body is a magnificent work of art. It has the ability to adapt to the many phases it will go through. Understanding the various stages and the experiences that are common can help you to better anticipate changes that may impact you and equip you with the knowledge to better care for your health.

PRE PREGNANCY: KNOW YOUR OWN BODY

Pregnancy is not the path for everyone. For those of us who do plan to undergo this stage, however, it is important to prepare ourselves in both mind and body. This starts with actually understanding the parts of us that will be actively involved with creating new life. In this section, we will explore just that, from the products we use in our daily routines, to the lesser-known pelvic organ. It is all about preparation! Our bodies are amazing, but they do not have to be mysterious.

Hygiene

No one wants to talk about it so guess what—you are about to read an entire chapter on it. How clean is your vagina?

Vaginal hygiene is a subject shrouded in misinformation and hidden behind centuries of patriarchal embarrassment. We have stuck things up there that shouldn't be. We have douched with bleach and animal products that were clearly a mistake. We have even taken to steaming the downstairs like a pampered princess on occasion. Whatever the method may be, our attempts at keeping our vaginas happy and healthy over the course of human history are fraught with well-intentioned mistakes. Today we are going to learn exactly why those mistakes were made in the past and how we can finally give our vaginas the care that they actually need.

How Our Product Choices Affect Our Pelvic Health

Many people are awakening to the truth about what's in their food and how certain ingredients negatively affect their health at some point. It may be the moment you realize that fast food every other day is making you lethargic or when we finally decide that milkshakes are not worth defying your lactose intolerant diagnosis. Most of us, however, don't stop to consider the ingredients in the personal care products that grace our most delicate regions and how they might be affecting our pelvic health.

Like the food we eat, the most beneficial and health-promoting personal care products are made with non-toxic, natural ingredients that don't disrupt the body's natural chemistry. The more simple, the better. In recent years, many products have entered the market that seem to offer exactly that. Although many do deliver on their promise, some do not.

Do not allow clever marketing slogans or pretty pink packaging fool you. Certain brands of tampons, pads, personal lubricants, wipes, deodorizers, and powders can negatively affect your pelvic health despite their buzzword packaging. Here is how to look past the words on the label and actually discern what products are actually good for your vagina.

Like many products in the health and beauty industry, the products we use on or near our nether regions can be full of junk (no pun intended). Using chemical-laden products on our pelvic area can lead to irritation, yeast infections, pelvic pain, allergic reactions, dryness—at a minimum. Each ingredient and additive carries with it a risk, and on a personal level, this should always be considered.

There can be far worse consequences than surface-level irritation, however. Exposure to endocrine-disrupting chemicals (or EDCs) found in many products can interfere with the normal function of the hormonal system and can contribute to an array of negative health impacts, including reproductive toxicity, endometriosis, ovulation disorders, and even an increased risk of cancer.

This is serious stuff, especially considering that the skin surrounding the genital area is thin and more permeable than skin covering the rest of the body, meaning harmful byproducts can be more easily absorbed. In fact, researchers from one study estimated that exposure to EDCs from menstrual products is at least ten times higher than the estimated absorption rates through the skin on other parts of the body.[3] Yikes.

In general, you need to be on the lookout for harmful chemicals in any feminine hygiene or personal care products including tampons, pads, period underwear, douches, sprays, washes, wipes, powders, or anything else that comes into contact with your pelvic region. If it touches your vagina in any capacity, give it a good, long side-eye. Now, this is where things get a little dicey. The FDA doesn't require companies to test for all harmful chemicals, nor do they require companies to disclose the presence of all chemicals used in these products. Given the widespread use of these products, this is a real concern. However, many of these harmful chemicals are listed on ingredient labels so always check the label before purchasing it.

What should you avoid? Well, there's a whole list, but we can focus on the worst offenders for now: phthalates and parabens. Phthalates are a group of plasticizer chemicals while parabens are most commonly used as a preservative. These two poisons, and many others, hide under hard-to-spell, complicated names. To make it more simple, never buy a product with the following ingredients:

- Benzethonium Chloride
- Benzocaine
- Butylparaben
- D&C Red 33
- Diazolidinyl Urea
- Dioxins and Furans
- DMDM Hydantoin
- Ethylparaben
- Ext. Violet 2
- FD&C Yellow No. 5
- "Fragrance"
- Methylchloroisothiazolinone
- Methylisothiazolinone
- Methylparaben
- Menthol
- Octoxynol 9
- Polyoxymethylene Urea
- Propylparaben
- Quaternium-15
- Sodium Hypochlorite
- 2-Bromo-2-Nitropropane-1, 3-Diol

Now, I know those words look like a bunch of gibberish, so I recommend printing out this list and always check it before making a product purchase. As mentioned above, the FDA isn't required to disclose the presence of all chemicals used in these types of products. Crazy, right?

Many organizations are working to do something about this, but in the meantime, here are some helpful tips for avoiding products that might contain hidden chemicals:

- Visit the list of "Hall of Shame" products and assess the products you may have in your home.
- Avoid the use of soaps, powders, and sprays. The vulva is self-cleaning and these products are unneeded and can actually create an environment where bacteria and fungal organisms will thrive, resulting in infections such as Bacteria Vaginosis (BV). A daily wash with clean, warm water should be sufficient to make you feel fresh.
- To the point above, reduce the number of personal care products you use in general, especially those that aren't medically necessary.
- If a product smells like a brand new shower curtain, run!
- If a product smells sickly sweet or artificial, pass!
- Use your intuition—if a product seems too cheap, it's probably low quality and filled with chemicals.
- Choose unscented products when available, especially in tampons and pads.
- Choose chlorine-free bleach or unbleached tampons and pads.
- Trade out your tampons for a menstrual cup made out of medical-grade silicone. It's reusable, non-toxic, and once you get the hang of it, a pretty nifty little product!

Your health matters. Toxic chemicals have no business hanging out "down there" and now that you know what to look out for, you can be more mindful of choosing pelvic-friendly products. You have a choice in which products you put on your body, so be your own advocate and choose wisely; your body deserves it.

THE ORGAN YOU DON'T KNOW YOU HAVE: FASCIA

News flash: your skin is NOT your largest organ! If you have never heard of fascia, you are not alone. Very few people are aware that there is a tissue that covers more of you than your skin, and that it can be the source of many problems and issues you may be facing in your daily life. Let's explore, together, what fascia is in the context of your body and how it can be affecting you everywhere, from the strange tingling in your feet to the tension headaches in your skull.

Fascia is a thin layer of connective tissue that lays over your muscles and extends all the way down to the cellular level of the body. It covers each organ, nerve, muscle, bone, and vein. The entirety of fascia is called the fascial system and when fascia is restricted it is often referred to as "the straight jacket." This epithet is derived from the fact that there is not a square inch of your body that does not have an overlay of fascial tissue. So, when your fascia cannot move freely, it is effectively binding you to your body. It becomes a trap that you cannot escape. In short, from the tip-top of your head to the bottom of your toes, fascia covers your entire being. The very basis of myofascial release (MFR) is identifying and treating restrictions within the little-known tissue called fascia.

This interesting part of your anatomy is composed of two types of fibers: collagenous fibers, which are very tough and have little stretchability; and elastic fibers, which are stretchable. It lies over your muscles and goes all the way down to the cellular level without interruption. It is considered to be a major system and organ known as the "interstitia." The interstitia is the only system that surrounds and invades every other tissue and organ of the body, including nerves, vessels, muscles, and bones. Interestingly, fascia is denser in some areas than others, depending on where in the body it is located.

My favorite analogy when explaining fascia is that of an orange. When we peel an orange, it easily separates into slices that are divided by a sturdy, transparent tissue. The tissue in the orange sections is similar to the fascia under our skin. The slices of oranges are held together under the thick, outer skin by a thin, white layer of pith, which is analogous to the superficial fascial layers that run throughout our bodies. In the very center of the orange there is a long, white center that keeps the orange connected and intact until it's pulled off or the slices are physically separated. This center connector is much like the deeper fascial layer beneath our skin. These deeper fascial layers hold our muscles and organs apart from one another, yet simultaneously hold them together in the same layer underneath the skin.

This extensive tissue serves multiple important functions as well, including the stabilization and connection of your various muscles and other tissues. If you were to peek beneath your skin, you would see it working constantly to keep you moving and functioning properly. Because of the overreaching nature of your fascial system, when damage occurs there is a long string of consequences throughout your many other systems. It is vulnerable for the exact reason it is so very strong: it is everywhere. Functionally, fascia allows the body to resist mechanical stresses, both internally and externally. It also provides a sliding and gliding environment for muscles, suspends organs in their proper place, transmits movement from muscles to the bones they are attached to, and provides a supportive and movable wrapping for nerves and blood vessels as they pass through and between muscles.

Of course, if fascia is not acting and reacting properly, you can begin to experience disorders of any one of these functions. When healthy, fascia is structured in a way that looks relaxed and wavy in configuration. It should be able to move and change with the rest of the body easily and without resistance. If an injury occurs and the physicality of fascia is altered through trauma, emotional or physical, it loses the pliable characteristics that are so very important to its function.

The fascia can "bunch up" when patterns are broken and over-adjusting occurs at the point of damage. When this happens, the layers of fascia are no longer uniform and can instead form knots, similar to those in a piece of lumber. These knots eventually restrict motion and can render certain movements impossible. This is when you see and feel fascia change in a noticeable way. It can feel hot, hard or tender, and rigid. Dehydrated, the tissues no longer glide along each other easily; it becomes more like beef jerky, immobile and tough. Fascial malfunction will begin to become more and more evident as the fascia is pulled tight or stretched beyond its abilities in places where it was not meant to stretch at all. This results in tissue restriction, decreased mobility, and ultimately, pain.

The main instigator of these irregularities is trauma. For our purposes, the term "trauma" describes events such as surgery, accidents, injury, repetitive activities, stress, and postural patterns. At the point of injury or trauma, fibers of the fascia become restricted and in turn, prevent fluid from passing through the fascial system the way that it should, as described above. This produces an incredible amount of tensile pressure. We talk a lot about how fascia is integral in all parts of our body. Our brain is no exception. Dura, or the specific fascia that encompasses the brain and adjoining central nervous system, has an important job. When healthy, the dura keeps the flow of oxygen to our cells and neurotransmitters unimpeded, and detoxes within those areas. As expected, when those functions are disrupted by pressure or injury, you are left with physiological illness, depression, anxiety, and nerve pain. Due to the overarching importance of the dura, some speculate that this also triggers our fight-or-flight response.

Keeping all of this in mind, let's explore the physicality behind this phenomenon. For example, Gerald H. Pollack, PhD at the University of Washington, provided a comprehensive study that probed into the specialized method that fluid moves through the fascial system, and why the restriction of fluid through the system is so damaging in his book, *The Fourth Phase of Water: Beyond Solid, Liquid and Vapor* (2014).

Dr. Pollack discovered that, despite the common conception that water exists in three states of matter (liquid, ice, and vapor), there is actually a fourth option: liquid crystal. Liquid crystal has character-istics of both a solid and a liquid, and has the capability to change. Fascia's properties are very similar to that of liquid crystal, making them almost synonymous, and thus there is a direct scientific connec-tion.[4] Pressure and restriction of fluid will cause pain. This pain, while often immense, is not something that will be evident in X-rays or MRI tests. As a result, many patients who experience pain that cannot be explained by an obvious injury through imaging are often overlooked by medical practitioners who do not have training in MFR. The pain then remains unchecked and untreated. Misdiagnosis runs rampant within the medical community pertaining to the particular subject of myofascial pain.

To further exacerbate this issue within pain management, the point of discomfort that a patient may be experiencing is often far from the true location of the fascial damage. Fluid restriction and points of stress can, and very often, affect the entire body. We likened fascia to a web for a reason. For example, patients may identify pain in their right shoulder when they are actually experiencing fascial abnormality at a surgery site on their back that had been operated on many years before.

The most simple way to illustrate the reasoning behind all of this is in the way Dr. Pollack himself describes fascia. According to him, we are not simply covered by fascia, we are in fact, "fascial beings."[4] It is a matrix, and by its very nature, adapts to us at the same time that we change because of it. There is no end to the immersive influence it has over us and all functions that make our lives possible. For many, many years physical therapists, like John F. Barnes, who knew this to be true, were invalidated by faulty and insufficient research. The issue was that we did not have accurate modeling of the human body when healthy and alive. Dr. Jean- Claude Guimberteau, a French hand and plastic surgeon, remedied this when in 2005 he updated the model of human anatomy through his groundbreaking research.[5]

With visual evidence, he was able to show exactly what fascial tissue actually looks like on a living human. This has become the irrefutable corroboration that John F. Barnes and Dr. Pollack needed to show that fascia is a completely integrated part of the body. Damage to fascia is much harder to remedy than a topical injury because of the static state of the tissue, even if it is identified and diagnosed. No amount of stretching, heating, icing, or exercise will lessen pain that stems from fascial damage because those conventional methods of pain alleviation do not address the source of the injury. Because of this, it can be the cause of chronic pain. Your chronic pain is present for a reason. Thanks to the researchers and physical therapists who have dedicated their lives to the study of fascia, you have a chance of not only identifying the reason for it, but also a treatment. Myofascial release has been built on this fact, now it is up to the patient to utilize it.

The Fascial Pelvis

The word "pelvis" originates from the Latin word for "basin." This is a fitting term, as a basin's most basic function is to hold fluids. Trauma and inflammatory responses tend to dehydrate ground substance within the fascial system, an issue for organisms like you and I, who are 70% fluid. In other words, when our basin runs dry, we begin to experience pain. You may be surprised that pelvic health is important in both men and women and can be treated in similar ways. Due to the nature of the pelvic floor, the way that the layers of muscle are surrounded by fascia, a balance of stability in relation to mobility is needed for it to function properly. It needs to be pliable in order to allow for expulsion as well as flexible for reproductive functions. The muscle tone should be adequate in order to provide stability, while not sacrificing the elasticity. A therapist can assess if deficiency in either is the cause of unexplained pain by determining if the patient requires stretching and relaxation in order to maximize mobility, or if strengthening of the muscle to promote support is needed. The true goal of treatment should focus on balancing the pelvis in order to create stability for the rest of the skeletal structure. Keeping this in mind, let's imagine that a patient is complaining of pain radiating from internal organs, such as the stomach or bladder, with no discernible cause. Traditional therapies may write it off and the patient could be prescribed pain medication as a temporary fix. Instead, I propose that there could be an abdominal scar from a cesarean section surgery that is putting pressure on the bladder and contributing to lumbar back pain, or hypertonus or trigger points in the abdominal muscles that have manifested itself in the pelvic area. It could also be piriformis syndrome, wherein the sciatic nerve and obturator internus form a sandwich and a sciatic nerve is being impinged upon; usually they all stem back to pelvic imbalance as the origin. These issues can be treated effectively with myofascial release therapy. In a more extreme example, let's say that a patient is experiencing painful intercourse, impotence, or incontinence. They could also have some discomfort while sitting. They could very well be suffering from pudendal nerve entrapment, which is a type of chronic pelvic pain caused by the compression of the pudendal nerve due to tightened fascia, muscles, or internal adhesions.

Our bodies are covered in nerve receptors. Certain areas have many more than the rest. The autonomic lumbosacral nerve plexus is one such cluster in your gut. Some actually refer to the gut as your second brain due to this fact. It provides hammock-like support for organs in the pelvic diaphragm, such as the intestines. If fascia is restricted, it won't just affect the vertebra (lumbar/sacrum/discs), it can also affect the function of our organs, causing problems with urination, bowel function, and digestion.

By providing gentle, sustained, hands-on compression and stretching into the areas of fascial restriction, a MFR therapist can restore the necessary slack to the system to take the pressure off of the pudendal nerve and surrounding structures that may be far away from the pelvic region. This helps to eliminate pain and improve the ability to sit, engage in intercourse, and maintain continence. As mentioned above, trauma is one of the main ways our fascial system becomes dehydrated of the fluid it is composed of, which results in pain, decreased motion, and compensation from other body joints, muscles, and tissue. Birth is the baby's first trauma and it's also a major trauma to your body, Mama. As a pelvic health specialist, authentic John Barnes Myofascial Release is one of the many techniques I utilize to help treat the prenatal and postpartum body. It is highly effective and beneficial to helping restore proper body alignment, reducing pain, and improving the tissue restrictions that birth causes. It is also highly effective in treating scar tissue both in the pelvic floor and along the C-section if you had one.

Fascia is a unique organ that should be more widely acknowledged. In women, it plays a huge role in your health from pregnancy and beyond. As you enter the newest stage of your life, remember to take this building block of your anatomy into account and treat it as you would any other part—with care, kindness, and understanding.

WHAT YOU SHOULD KNOW ABOUT YOUR PELVIC FLOOR: PRE-PREGNANCY & DURING PREGNANCY

Pregnancy is one of the most beautiful times of a person's life. It is both exciting and full of responsibility. Pregnancy is a life-changing experience, especially for women, because our bodies undergo significant changes during pregnancy and after childbirth. If you've ever been pregnant, more than likely, you have had your elders and friends telling you to eat healthily, stay happy, exercise, and so much more.

This is because every stage of pregnancy, along with its beautiful moments, has its issues and concerns. In fact, studies also suggest that 8% of all pregnancies involve complications.[6] And if you are not prepared to tackle them, sadly, this beautiful experience can become life-threatening! Now is the time to begin preparing at the ground floor—the pelvic floor that is.

What is the Pelvic Floor?

The layers of muscles, connective tissues, and ligaments surrounding the rectum and vagina make up our pelvic floor. These layers of muscles stretch between our pubic area and tailbone, supporting our abdominal organs, including the uterus, bladder, and bowel. The healthy functioning of these muscles is crucial for maintaining the pregnancy, defecation, urination, vaginal intercourse, childbirth, and several other processes.

Nature has designed the pelvic floor with ligaments allowing it to stretch under pressure to provide adequate support and bounce back after childbirth. It works to promote healthy bowels and significant bladder control. If our pelvic floor doesn't work properly and is unhealthy, it can cause discomfort during urination and sexual intercourse and lead to miscarriages, birth defects, and post-pregnancy disorders. In some cases, if a woman is at risk of losing her pregnancy due to a weak pelvic floor, she is placed on strict bed rest for the remainder of her pregnancy duration.

Why is Pelvic Floor Health Essential for Pregnancy?

The health of your pelvic floor is very vital before, after, and during pregnancy. The strain of carrying a child growing inside our bodies can be damaging for the pelvic floor muscles. This is because the pelvic floor has to make room for the baby, and as such, the pelvic floor stretches its muscles to accommodate our little one. As the baby grows, these pelvic floor muscles expand even further and get weighed down, putting them at risk of becoming weakened and strained and putting excess pressure on our organs.

If your pelvic floor is already healthy, these muscles will be strong enough to withstand the stretching and weight, and the damage they endure will be very minimal. However, an unhealthy or weak pelvic floor encountering such strain can cause weaker muscles and damage during pregnancy.

Also, a healthy pelvic floor ensures that we are readily equipped for labor and delivery. Delivery is likely to be less risky and strenuous, which means less stress for both the mother and baby, if you have a healthy pelvic floor. If you have a vaginal delivery or a C-section, the layers of muscles in the pelvic floor experience a bit of straining and stretching. If the pelvic floor is healthy enough, the muscles will return to their optimal level of functioning and location soon thereafter, so we are likely to recover faster after the delivery. Otherwise, if the pelvic muscles were not in the best shape going into the labor and delivery process, it means post-delivery pelvic complications can be expected.

A healthier pelvic floor is a stronger pelvic floor and that makes it easier for us to control our bladder and rectum during and after pregnancy. A lack of bladder control during pregnancy is observed most frequently during the second and third trimesters. This is because our pelvic floor is weak, so we cannot squeeze the muscles as required to stop urine from evading the bladder. In the worst-case scenario, a weak pelvic floor can cause pelvic organs to move out of their places into the vagina. When this occurs, it is diagnosed as pelvic organ prolapse, which is extremely painful. What happens is that our ligaments loosen up during pregnancy due to the production of hormones like oxytocin & relaxin. These ligaments are tissues that keep our organs in place, and when loosened, they can't hold onto them.[7] We will delve much more into this condition a bit later.

Signs of an Unhealthy Pelvic Floor

Now that we know the complications associated with a weakened pelvic floor, let's look for the signs to find out if ours is healthy or not. If it is healthy, that's great; we just need to keep doing whatever it is that we're doing. If not, it's not the end of the world. All we need to do is take a bit more care of our pelvic floor muscles.

Here are the more common signs and symptoms of an unhealthy pelvic floor:

- **Urinary incontinence:** If urine involuntarily exits the body during daily activities, like walking, coughing, laughing, etc., the pelvic floor may be weak.
- **Fecal incontinence:** If we uncontrollably pass stool during everyday activities for even a short time, it may be an indication that the pelvic floor is unhealthy.
- **Urinary and fecal retention:** This is another sign of a weakened pelvic floor when we have much difficulty emptying the bladder or rectum.
- **Painful sex:** Experiencing extreme pain during sexual intercourse is another sign of a weakened pelvic floor.
- If you see a bulge distended from the vagina or feel like the vagina is full or something is protruding from the vaginal opening, it can be an indication of pelvic organ prolapse.

Prevalence of Pelvic Floor Disorders

According to the National Health and Nutritional Examination Survey (NHANES), from 2005-2010, almost 8,000 women in the United States were found to experience symptoms of a pelvic disorder. What is even more shocking is that all of these women were non-pregnant.[8] Also, in the United Kingdom, 1 in 3 women experience bladder leakage caused by a weak pelvic floor. Another study investigating the prevalence of pelvic floor disorders in Australian women found that almost 48% of the women included in the study reported physiological strain in their pelvic floor during early and late pregnancy.[9]

In a community-based study that was conducted to assess the magnitude of pelvic floor disorders in Kersa district Eastern Ethiopia, it was determined that of the 3,432 women that participated in the study, 704 reported at least one type of pelvic floor disorder and 349 experienced two or more pelvic floor disorders. Additionally, the most common pelvic floor disorders included an over active bladder, pelvic organ prolapse, stress urinary and anal incontinence. The study also reported that more than two-thirds of the women with pelvic floor disorders reported having severe distress, but had never sought health care. This delay may have led to other complications and worsening of the conditions.[10]

A cross-sectional study conducted in 2019, which involved 346 participants, evidenced that pelvic floor disorders consisting of urinary incontinence, fecal incontinence, and pelvic organ prolapse is estimated to range between 12 and 42%, and symptoms can present as early as age 20.[11]

Researchers report that women fail to get medical attention due to several misconceptions about the pelvic floor conditions. In fact, a specific study revealed that 81% of women do not perceive urinary incontinence as abnormal and believe that pelvic floor disorders are a "natural part of childbirth and aging".[11]

These studies indicate that pelvic disorders are common among both pregnant and non-pregnant women. Also, healthcare providers from major hospitals in the US assert that a significant number of women have and are at risk of developing pelvic disorders.[8,9] This situation shows evidence of an alarming proportion in society and thus needs to be addressed immediately. Young women who are thinking of having a child are advised to prepare themselves first, including the pelvic floor. We should make sure that our pelvic floor is strong enough to carry and deliver our babies without the worry of complications. It will not only be beneficial for the mother, but the baby also.

Pelvic Organ Prolapse

Pelvic floor physical therapy is a great option following surgeries such as hysterectomies, episiotomies, bladder surgeries, colorectal surgeries, or C-sections. When the muscles are cut during pelvic or abdominal surgery, it takes a period of healing before they are able to grow back together and regain their former strength. Following surgery, you might also notice that you have scar tissue and flexibility issues. Through exercises and manual therapy, pelvic floor physical therapy can help restore the function, strength, and mobility of your pelvic floor and core muscles.

This is evident through the treatment of our first condition. Pelvic organ prolapse occurs when one or more of your pelvic organs, such as your bladder, uterus, or rectum, descends into or even out of your vagina or its canal due to a loss of muscle and/or connective tissue support.

Symptoms can include a feeling of heaviness or pressure "down there," trouble fully emptying your bladder or having a bowel movement, or seeing a bulge of tissue coming out of your vaginal opening. I know that sounds scary, but there is help available if you know when to reach out. Through targeted exercises, stretches, and manual therapy techniques, physical therapy works to get the transverse abdominis or rib cage/diaphragm and pelvic floor working properly and strengthen the supporting core muscles. The best-case scenario is recognizing that you have pelvic organ prolapse and treating it with pelvic floor physical therapy to avoid surgery. Prolapse-safe exercises will typically focus on finding your transverse abdominis muscle (TRA), internal oblique, and rectus abdominis (RA) muscle and how to strengthen them. Your pelvic health therapist will also work with you to help you connect your breath and abdominals, improve your core activation in daily movement, and mobilize your pelvis for core control. The diaphragm and respiration have a significant influence on posture patterns and movement dysfunction.

We breathe approximately 20,000 times a day. By the time you're 50 years of age you have taken around 400 million breaths.[12] Often, during treatment, I will address how to properly engage the diaphragm muscles, as they are very closely connected to the pelvic floor and the rest of the body. We need to be able to find a neutral position where our rib cage and pelvis stack on top of each other to decrease compensation and improve our ability to restore movement options. Muscles in the neck and lumbar region often take up the slack if we are not breathing efficiently with our diaphragm.

How Pregnancy Changes the Pelvis

During pregnancy, the pelvic joint loosens to accommodate the fetus. This change begins around 10 weeks, so if a woman is planning to become pregnant, they must expect this. These pelvic joint movements will cause a pregnant woman to have pain and cramps. After delivery, the joints typically revert to normal at approximately 4-12 weeks post pregnancy.

Pelvic floor dysfunction is one condition that could affect women during pregnancy due to the nature of childbirth. If we experience prolonged labor, the use of instruments during delivery, such as forceps, may occur or the woman may receive a tear or incision (episiotomy). Approximately 50% of women endure pelvic pain during pregnancy. 8% of these women report pain that causes severe disability, while 25% describe experiencing severe pelvic girdle pain.[13,14]

How to Prepare the Pelvic Floor for Pregnancy

Preparing your pelvic floor is simple and essential. It is never too late to begin taking care of this unique part of your body, and the effects you will feel whether you are planning to become pregnant, are pregnant, or are postpartum are incredible.

Maintain a Healthy Lifestyle

First things first, adjust your lifestyle as much as possible. Give up on any unhealthy habits, such as bad eating habits, and switch to healthy ones. Make sure you have healthy body weight, and your BMI is normal. To check your BMI, Google standard weight as per your age and height and calculate your BMI. If it lies within the overweight or obese section, start a proper workout and healthy diet. Incorporate a significant portion of fruits and vegetables into your diet. Avoid fried and processed food.

If you are already pregnant, maintain a healthy weight gain. Ensure to get your caregiver's permission before you practice activities and exercises that cause your abdomen to bear pressure, especially if you are within your fourth or above month of pregnancy. If you are working in an office or at home, give yourself enough time to rest. Try to attend yoga classes for pregnant women. Regularly see a pelvic health physical therapist and explore the health of your pelvic floor.

Engage Yourself in Safe Pelvic Floor Exercise

Certain exercises strengthen your muscles, for example, Kegel exercise, pelvic tilts, bridges, etc. Try to practice these activities under expert guidance. I repeat, do not just follow YouTube and Facebook tutorials blindly. Contact a specialist physical therapist trained in women's health and ask for directives. Don't hesitate to ask questions to ensure that you fully understand your responsibilities and limitations. As pelvic exercises are sometimes very tricky, it might be problematic to know which muscles should be squeezed and when. That's why we have the experts to train us to do them the right way as instructed. If you are having a problem while exercising or experience any kind of pain, contact your doctor or specialist therapist immediately.

The five most recommended exercises for strengthening the muscles of the pelvic floor include:

- Kegels
- Pelvic tilts
- Squats
- Split tabletop
- Bird dog

Be cautious if you are given an absolute answer like never lift, squat, or jump. While you can check how to perform these exercises on the Internet, it is imperative you contact a specialist women's health physical therapist to assess if they are appropriate for you now or if you need some preventative work prior to strengthening your pelvic floor. Again, I say this with the utmost caution, do not just do Kegels and start strengthening your pelvic floor if you don't know whether or not you have a strength issue or an issue with tissue tightness. More harm will be done by blindly strengthening if it is not what you truly need. You should not be curating your plan of care off the Internet. You deserve to work with a provider as you deserve formula education and a proper assessment as well as a plan of care. Also, remember, the pelvic floor muscles are not, I repeat, are not what pushes the baby out of the vaginal canal, it's the uterus that does that job!

Eat Foods That Strengthen Your Pelvic Floor

A healthy diet is one of the safest ways to escape any kind of health complications. So, you should adopt a healthy diet for strengthening your pelvic floor. Water, bananas, oily fish, avocados, and eggs are five of the best foods that aid in supporting a weak pelvic floor. The nutrients in these food items can provide you with adequate nutrition to promote healthy muscle growth. Plus, their low-fat content will keep you away from unnecessary weight gain.

BACK PAIN BEFORE, DURING, AND AFTER PREGNANCY

I t is not uncommon for women to complain of back pain during pregnancy and after birth. About 50% to 75% of all pregnant women suffer back pain at some point during pregnancy.[14] The extra weight resulting from the increased body weight during the latter stages of pregnancy, can easily be pointed as the cause of such back pains. So, what can be the cause of back pains during early parts of the pregnancy and the back pains felt even after delivery?

The most obvious answer is that women gain weight during pregnancy, typically between 25-35 pounds. The spine is then tasked with supporting the extra weight of the baby and the uterus, a job it is not used to doing. The increase in weight in these structures can begin to irritate nerves in the low back, causing pain down one or both legs and sometimes even into the feet and toes. If you have never suffered from low back pain prior to pregnancy, your core muscles could simply not be strong enough to support the additional weight necessary to grow a baby. For many women, back pain will subside once the baby is born.

Unfortunately, however, one in three women will continue to experience symptoms of low back pain up to one year postpartum.[15]

The life changes that occur with having a baby are significant and the stress of having back pain only adds another layer of complexity to life with a new baby. Be proactive. Physical therapy can be a safe and effective treatment to provide the necessary tools in order to manage and eradicate your symptoms so that your time and energy can be focused on the new life you have created. Physical therapy can also be a useful treatment to facilitate a smoother pregnancy and birth.

A study published in 2014, in the *Journal of Orthopedic and Sports Physical Therapy*, examined the most effective treatments for women experiencing low back pain during pregnancy.[16] Although we will explore several different treatment options here, research has found the most effective therapy to be exercise and patient education. Specifically, patient education surrounding activity modification and lifestyle changes.[17] If you are experiencing low back pain with pregnancy, here are several options to consider discussing with your health care provider and physical therapist.

Specific Exercise: These are exercises prescribed by your therapist including (but are not limited to) strengthening of the pelvic floor, core, and posture muscles. An exercise program tailored directly to your needs and muscle imbalances, while working closely with your therapist, will ensure you are getting the best care for your specific condition. This may also include education on things you should *not* be doing during episodes of pain.

Perineal Massage: This type of massage involves the gentle stretching and massaging of the skin between the anus and vagina (perineum) during the last few weeks of pregnancy. This treatment has been shown to reduce the episode of perineal tears during birth. Perineal massage also prepares you for the pressure and stretching that occurs when the baby's head crowns and enables you to relax, leading to a quicker delivery.

SI Belt: The pelvic girdle is a region of ligaments and muscles where the ilium (our hip bone) and the sacrum meet to form three joints at the base of the spine. In order for these bones to have some movement when we walk, muscles and ligaments must work to stabilize them. Important muscles that aid in stabilization of the pelvic girdle include the transverse abdominis, psoas major, multifidi, and the pelvic floor muscles. During pregnancy these muscles can become less efficient due to increased loads placed upon them. When exercise alone is not enough to increase stabilization in this region, a sacroiliac belt may be used to help stabilize the lower back.

On the other hand, it is important to keep in mind treatments that are contraindicated, aka not safe. There should be no modalities used during physical therapy. Ultrasound and ESTIM, two commonly used passive modalities in physical therapy clinics, are contraindicated during pregnancy. Ultrasound, a therapeutic modality used for the deep heating of tissues through high-frequency sound pulses can expose the fetus and result in overheating. ESTIM should also be avoided early in pregnancy due to its potential to cause abortion. The effects of TENS on a developing fetus is uncertain and clinicians should use extra caution when considering potential risk vs. benefit for application to distant sites (non-abdominal areas).

Many women are nervous to exercise during pregnancy, but research has shown it is not only safe and healthy for the expecting mom and baby, but it can also help to reduce the length of labor and delivery and cause less painful contractions.[18]

Back pains in pregnant women typically occur where the pelvis meets the spine, at the sacroiliac joint. This can be the result of several factors. Postural and natural anatomic changes bring about mechanical challenges to the lower back and other parts of the musculoskeletal system. These challenges cause the lumbar spine to increase its C-shaped curvature, causing extra strain on the ligaments, muscles, and lumbar joints. Consequently, the psoas muscle in the hip gets shortened and is not able to adequately stabilize the spine. These actions increase lower back pain and sciatica symptoms (in some instances). Some women may also experience pelvic pains.

Causes:

Hormonal changes. During pregnancy, women produce the hormone, relaxin. Relaxin makes the ligaments in the pelvic region relax and causes the joints to become loose to allow for a smooth delivery of the baby. Sometimes, relaxin causes the ligaments that support the spine to relax as well, causing back pains.

Posture changes. Pregnant women experience a shift in their center of gravity. This shift adjusts their posture and movement, leading to strain or back pains.

Weight gain. The extra weight pregnant women put on causes their spine to support more weight. Aside from the spine, blood vessels and nerves in the back and pelvis take some of this pressure. The pressure on the spine, blood vessels, and nerves result in lower back pains.

Muscle Separation. Sometimes when the womb expands, the rectal muscles separate along the center seam. This can worsen back pain.

Stress. Emotional stress can also cause muscle tension, which may be felt as back pain.

Medical history. Women with a history of back pains and pre-existing lower back disorders may experience it during pregnancy.

Age. Women considered to be younger or older than the ideal pregnancy age range are more likely to develop lower back pains during pregnancy.

Treatment

- Wear low–heeled shoes or footwear to allow for an even distribution of your body weight.
- Do not lift heavy objects. If you need to pick something, ask for help. Otherwise, bend your knees and keep your back straight whenever you want to pick or lift something; do not bend over.
- Always try to keep things balanced. For instance, when you go shopping, distribute the items in two bags and carry with both hands to keep balance.
- Avoid locking your knees.
- Use a good and proper mattress to enhance a good posture when sleeping. You may sleep on your side with a pillow between your knees, behind your back, and under your abdomen to reduce stress on your spine.
- Regular exercise boosts flexibility and strengthens muscles. It helps reduce stress on the spine. As a pregnant woman, not all exercises are safe for you. You can try walking, stationary cycling, and other exercises recommended to you by your physical therapist or doctor.
- Stand every 20 minutes and try to avoid sitting for prolonged hours. This will help promote blood flow as well as give your spine and hips a rest. Increased sitting increases the force through the spine, which can lead to back pain, hip pain and pelvic pain. You can reduce these risks by standing every 20 minutes.
- Use maternity support pillows when sitting. In the absence of a pillow, keep your back straight. Slouching will strain your spine.
- Sleep with a body pillow between your legs to keep your spine aligned, especially as your pelvis begins to widen. This will help

reduce low back tension as it decreases the amount of twisting at your lower spine.

- Avoid sitting cross legged. Your spine isn't designed to turn or twist. Sitting cross legged does just that. Your joints have increased laxity during pregnancy, which puts you at an increased risk of injury during pregnancy; even just the feet being crossed causes your pelvis and spine to be twisted, which stresses the joints and muscles and leads to an experience of unwanted stresses that leave you vulnerable to injury.

Postpartum Back Pain

Some women still suffer lower pains even after delivery. Generally, the pain should go away within six months after delivery, but it may endure in some (about a third) women for up to a year or more.

Causes

- Hormones: The pregnancy hormones are still to blame. It takes up to six months for the high pregnancy hormone levels to fall back to normal. The pains should recede as the body itself also recovers from the pregnancy within a few months—in addition to the drop in hormone level.
- Strained abdominal muscles: The strained muscles you develop as a result of pushing in the delivery room, or from C-section, affect your posture, putting some strain on your spine.
- Physical activity: Lifting your baby the wrong way, bending, and other physical activities that affect your body posture can also play a part.

Treatment

- **Exercise.** Walking and yoga are good exercises for women who have undergone either a normal delivery or a C-section. It's important as the pelvis stretches and your ribs move that you take time to support the changing length of the muscles. Stretching and strengthening can help you accomplish this. Healthy muscles are able to contract and relax and as your body changes it's important to nurture these changes. Pilates and even Barre are helpful if you want to avoid pregnancy-related pains.
- **Get physical therapy.** Both prenatal and postnatal back pains, as well as pelvic/hip pains, can be treated with physical therapy. Physical therapy is one of the most professional and advisable ways to combat back pain, especially when it is getting severe. A prenatal physical therapy evaluation is highly recommended to help you easily transition through each week of your pregnancy to the postpartum state.

I share with you the eight strategies and principles that you can do to help work for you. Some may work instantly; some may take time. There is no order to this, but they all work. These are strategies that were created through not just research, but through careful observation and experience. I have created this report because sometimes you just need these "small steps" to get you to the next step. Now my challenge to you is to try these strategies out. It won't take long, but it does take time to do some of these every day. I think you might be pleasantly surprised how much better you feel.

1. Stand on one leg or the OPPOSITE leg
   If you are like every human being on this planet, you are a righty or a lefty. Not just in the upper extremities, but in the lower

extremities as well. You subconsciously tend to lean on one leg OR you try to stand on two legs all the time. If you notice that, try standing on the opposite leg or try shifting to one leg. You'll be surprised how this can affect you.

2. Sit or sleep on the OTHER side

   Like point number one, being aware of these positions is sometimes the first thing to do. Just like when you are addicted to something. The first step is to be aware. Check if you tend to cross your legs one way a lot or you tend to sleep on one side all the time. Just switch it up and give that other hip a BREAK!

3. Stop squeezing your a**

   Glute/butt strengthening exercises are very popular nowadays if you follow any fitness/exercise social media. There is a place and time for them. However, if you've been doing a ton of glute exercises without relief, try taking a break and relax your gluteal region.

4. Avoid stretching your hamstrings

   Yes, I did say it. For now, hold off on stretching your hamstrings. You'll be surprised how many people keep stretching their hamstrings because they feel "tight." Sometimes they are feeling tight possibly due to other reasons, such as weakness, poor core stability, OR even just stress. If you are a person that has been stretching hamstrings without relief, hold off stretching them and see where it takes you.

5. Stay away from wearing heels

   Heels are great for fashion, but poor for function. When you have elevated heels, it tends to put your hip and pelvis in a poor position. If you do this for too long, your body might not know how to put that hip and pelvis back into place when you don't wear your heels. HINT HINT: The ankle/feet can affect the hips and lower back.

6. Strengthen your hamstrings

   We are upright bipedal mammals for a reason. Your back muscles help you keep upright, but often they are on too much. The hamstrings help us stay upright too. Try doing some hamstring exercises without over tensing your face/body and see how things feel.

7. Get a full evaluation from a health care professional

   Whether it is with a chiropractor, physical therapist, or athletic trainer who has a medical professional that you trust to assess you. It's difficult to objectively assess yourself when you are in pain. An objective assessment from an expert will go a long way for you.

8. Get assessed by a pelvic floor/women's health PT

   This is one of the most important things you could do for yourself before, during, and after pregnancy. Your body is about to or has gone through significant changes in space and against gravity and getting assessed and treated by a women's health specialist is the fastest way to ease back pain. Most often, exercises alone are not nearly enough to address the root cause of the problem. During pregnancy, it's common for joints to become loose, stiff, or even locked and the only way to help loosen them is by hand.

HOW TO MAKE YOUR PELVIC FLOOR WORK FOR YOU

Though it may not get the attention and recognition as other parts of your anatomy, like your brain or even your arms, there is a lot happening in the bony bowl defined by your hip bones, pubic bone, and sacrum. When it functions properly, your pelvic floor provides support for your pelvic organs, helps you stand, maintains control of your bladder, and bowel function, and is responsible for healthy sexual activity. In other words, it's something you *really* want to work well. However, things can go awry in your pelvic floor for a variety of reasons, leading to painful and disruptive symptoms. This is not uncommon—a 2008 study by the *Journal of the American Medical Association* shows evidence that roughly one-quarter of US women are affected by pelvic floor disorders.[19] Yet, we rarely name our sickness.

It is unfortunate that despite the high number of those suffering, awareness is so quiescent. Many women feel embarrassed about the symptoms they are experiencing, don't know where to go for help, or don't even realize that their symptoms are not normal. It is not an easy subject to talk about and can conjure up quite a bit of embarrassment for women, but that is exactly why it is so important. When we can talk about it candidly, we can also talk about treatment.

Everyone knows that physical therapy can be used to rehab an ankle or neck, but few people are aware that physical therapy can also play a major role in recovery from a variety of pelvic floor conditions. We are about to discuss how the proper use of pelvic physical therapy can help with pelvic or abdominal surgery, pelvic organ prolapse, stress incontinence, and diastasis recti. These three conditions are the most common faced by women today.

It is important to note that caring for your pelvic floor is not something that should only be done *after* you notice a problem. **Women should begin thinking about their pelvic health before they become pregnant or before they start having signs and symptoms of pelvic dysfunction.** Through targeted work, we have the power to prevent— or greatly minimize— potential pelvic issues and encourage faster, smoother recovery from pelvic dysfunction, surgeries, and childbirth. Additionally, engaging in pelvic floor therapy before and during pregnancy can facilitate an easier vaginal delivery and recovery. It is never too early or late to start working on your pelvic floor health and core strength.

Diastasis Recti

Our next condition can sound equally as scary, but can be easily treated. After you come home from delivering your beautiful baby, you might be wondering what in the world happened to your abdominal muscles. The answer is diastasis recti (also known as DRA). This condition occurs when the linea alba, a connective tissue sheet that joins together the two sides of the rectus abdominis muscle, widens and thins. This creates a separation of these muscles called a diastasis. Mom translation? It's that annoying post-baby stomach pooch that just won't seem to go away.

The pregnancy hormones surging through your body relaxes connective tissue in order to allow the growth your body needs during the pregnancy. As this hormone increases, so does your tissue's flexibility. The fascia, linea alba, begins to stretch and thin and when you finally give birth and once you no longer need this flexibility, your muscles are meant to grow back together. Unfortunately, 33% of women do not heal properly on their own within the 6-8 weeks that most doctors give you to be declared healed and ready for regular activity. That is not to say most will not heal on their own eventually—40% of women's abdominal muscles grow back together by 6 months postpartum and 32% after 12 months.[20]

There are some factors that can make it more likely that you will suffer from this dysfunction, such as having a petite build, carrying multiples, and having multiple full-term pregnancies. You may also be more at risk if your pregnancy occurs at a later stage in life, have poor muscle tone before pregnancy and during, or, lastly, have a swayback posture. When pregnancy is the cause of DRA, baby size and weight gain do not affect the severity of a diastasis, as is commonly thought.

Since transverse abdominis tightness and weakness contributes to diastasis and belly distention as well as back tightness, you can suffer from DRA without pregnancy as well. The frequent or rapid change in weight, obesity, genetics, and poor training technique when lifting have all been shown to cause this condition. It is not as common, but still important to note.

Preventing DRA during pregnancy is tricky. There are many factors that we cannot always control. However, there are steps we can take to lessen our risk. Prevention is always superior to after-treatment, after all. As a physical therapist, I attack the condition on four levels: education, posture training, bracing, and exercise.

Education is our first step because when you know what is going on with you internally, you can make external changes that will help. A professional can educate you on the most appropriate way to use your treatment as well as point you in the right direction when other symptoms present. Over time and as you become more informed, you learn how to best care for your body.

Much of your symptoms may be stemming from the way you carry yourself, at least physically. When you have poor posture, you are not engaging your deep core muscles correctly. Even the way you breathe comes right back to how you sit, walk, and stand. It is a basic building block that too often gets ignored even though it is the number one priority for our body! Most DR patients do not have good lateral expansion with their breathing. This is often one of the first things I address when treating a patient who is suffering from DR.

Bracing is a later treatment option. A physical therapist may recommend taping or using braces around your core during your recovery period if they feel it is appropriate. This gives your abdominal muscles the support they need to achieve good posture and facilitate healing.

The most accessible level is exercise. This can be a preventative measure as well. Strengthening your core muscles before pregnancy gives them the support and strength they will need as they go through the changes that will come later. When exercising your core focus on the following muscle groups: external abdominal oblique, internal abdominal oblique, rectus abdominis, transversus abdominis.

Good exercises to strengthen these muscles include a pelvic tilt with a crunch on a balance ball, modified push ups, hip circles on a balance ball, cat pose, opposite arm and leg extension, and bridge stability on a ball. Ideally, you should work with a physical therapist who can evaluate you and design a prenatal fitness program that addresses your particular weaknesses. They can help you not only strengthen your core, but also maintain that strength when it matters.

Instead of only focusing on typical abdominal exercises, a physical therapist can guide you in the appropriate way to actually engage your deeper layers of the abdominals called the transverse abdominal muscle. A pelvic physical therapist is also able to work with you on daily tasks that so often become unexpected sources of pain and injury. From getting out of bed to lifting your baby, you have the opportunity to protect your physical well-being when you know exactly why and how your body works.

In our society, a new mother's crowning achievement is walking away from the hospital at their pre-pregnancy weight. In fact, the focus on losing baby weight quickly and almost obsessively extends to the medical community. Most training on post-birth care focuses on how to get women back into the gym. As I have seen in my own clinic, this leads to the misconception that it is natural and expected to jump back into regular routines with little attention paid to your physical well-being.

Once you have given birth, you will forever be postpartum. Your body has entered a new and exciting phase. Taking care of it means embracing this fact. You are unique and you are beautiful at each stage of your life. Treat your body with kindness wherever you find yourself.

Your pelvic floor is your best friend when addressing all four of these dysfunctions. It is a part of your inner core as it is located at the floor of your pelvis. This part of your anatomy is what holds your baby for the full nine months and because of that, even if you deliver via C-section, it has been through quite the ordeal. Rehabbing the pelvic floor will aid in your overall recovery more than any amount of crunches or leg lifts.

Pelvic floor muscle contractions, or Kegels, are exercises you can do to begin strengthening your pelvic floor. Like all exercises, doing them properly means the difference between injuring yourself further or gaining strength so doing so under the guidance of a professional is preferable. If this is not possible, being informed on the proper technique and being purposeful in your movements is of the utmost importance.

Kegels are most beneficial when used during exhalation. Learning to sync your diaphragmatic breathing and pelvic floor contractions will promote proper stability throughout your entire inner core. A physical therapist who specializes in the pelvic floor is trained to do an internal and external assessment of these muscles in order to give you the right type of exercises to help your individual needs. Believe it or not, Kegels are not usually the first line of treatment for most women.

In tandem with physical exercise, one should also be addressing your body's nutritional needs. Vitamins C and A, and zinc are important for collagen regeneration and helping connective tissue fibers to become taut. Vitamin C can be found in fresh fruit and vegetables, such as red peppers, tomatoes, and kiwis. You can boost Vitamin A by eating carrots, sweet potatoes, and kale. Get zinc from nuts, seeds, and beans. Protein is also important in tissue healing. Include good protein with every meal. Some foods that are good sources of protein are grass-fed or organic meat, fish, nuts, and eggs.

Foods that are rich in iron help improve the oxygenation in your blood due to the fact that iron is a carrier of oxygen to the blood cells. Examples of iron-rich foods include beef, broccoli, and apricots. Alpha-linolenic acid (essential fatty acids) is another important component of your healing diet. It improves the body's absorption of fat-soluble vitamins, has a positive effect on immune response, and boosts energy. So, eat plenty of oily fish, seeds, nuts, avocados, and eggs. As you prepare meals, you can utilize oils, such as olive oil, coconut oil, grapeseed oil, and hemp oil, to ensure that you are meeting your dietary needs.

Staying hydrated is important as well. Water is crucial for detoxifying and hydrating connective tissue and for boosting circulation. You should be intaking about 11.5 cups or 2.7 liters of water[21] every day, adjusting for your activity level and other factors, of course.

Hypertonic Pelvic Floor

If you have hypertonic pelvic floor muscles, Kegels will make your symptoms worse. If you have an uncoordinated pelvic floor, you may not perform the Kegels correctly and this can cause further issues. I can't stress this highly enough—if you are not sure what to do, find a pelvic floor physical therapist in your area to perform a thorough pelvic floor internal examination to determine the root cause of your pelvic floor dysfunction. Are your muscles tight? Are your muscles uncoordinated? Are they actually, truly just weak (rare but can happen)? Chances are these symptoms will not just go away on their own. You deserve individualized treatment. You deserve to heal from these symptoms and to address the root cause of them for long-lasting relief.

Pelvic pain: Your pelvic muscles have gone through a lot during childbirth and putting your pelvic muscles under more strain when they're already weak is not a good idea. To minimize or avoid additional pelvic pain, try postnatal abdominal muscle bracing and pelvic floor exercises after six weeks to strengthen your muscles.

Painful intercourse: If you push your body to work out and do the things you could before you gave birth, you're heading down a dangerous path. Many women have been left with painful health conditions by trying to bounce back into shape too soon. From painful intercourse to suffering a prolapse, it's simply not worth the risks. I ask my weekly patients if they have resumed intercourse postpartum and more often than not they haven't and admit to feeling guilty about it.

Most women go on to further explain that they are nervous, tired, or admit to just not feeling like their usual self. I always tell them that they have every right to wait to resume intercourse until they feel ready. So much has changed since having sex prior to pregnancy. The pelvic floor and stomach muscles have been stretched and things are functioning a bit differently. Don't feel guilty or judged.

Your healthcare team (OBGYN, midwife, nurse practitioner, and your pelvic floor physical therapist) are not judging you. We are on your team and want you to be successful, so if things aren't feeling right, or you are nervous, see a pelvic floor physical therapist. It is common for your muscles to feel achy after the first attempt. The muscles haven't been used in that activity for a while. Similar to when you workout for the first time your leg/arm muscles can be crampy, so can the muscles in your lower abdomen and pelvic floor after sex. However, if it continues, see a pelvic floor physical therapist.

So, when you finally reach your 6-week postpartum check-up, rather than feel down about the number on the scale, and try to force yourself to work out, reward your body with plenty of fresh fruit and nutritious snacks. Your body has given you the greatest gift of all! So, respect it, care for it, and most of all, show it unconditional love.

The pelvic floor muscles are made up of several layers. The first layer of the pelvic floor muscles is the superficial layer: ischiocaavernosus, bulbocavernosus, superficial transverse perineum, external anal sphincter, and external urethral sphincter. They are all connected in one way or another. This group of muscles works to close their openings, prevent leakage, and tell the bladder when it is available to release urine.

These muscles are often unconditional and sometimes weakened in women. We should be able to control them consciously when we sit down to urinate and subconsciously when we cough, sneeze, laugh, run, jump, etc. However, sometimes that's not the case.

When women say they have "tried Kegels" and haven't seen a change in their leaking, I remind them it is not that simple. You see, the pelvic floor muscles need to move like other muscles in your body. They should contract or shorten like your arm does to pick something up and they should lengthen or relax. As women, we often forget the relaxation piece and then have increased symptoms of urgency/frequency. Working on lengthening the pelvic floor muscles can often be the most challenging part of retraining these muscles to improve symptoms.

Pelvic floor therapy is recommended as a first-line treatment for pelvic disorders for a reason. Proper physical therapy can prevent surgery in many cases and reduce the risk of associated injury. Try not to feel embarrassed if you're experiencing a pelvic floor disorder. Your pelvis is part of you and deserves the same care and treatment as any other part of your body. There's no need to suffer in silence—reach out to a pelvic floor physical therapist today and be on your way to a full recovery!

THE BENEFITS OF EXERCISE DURING PREGNANCY

Get moving, Mama! Seriously, I know it feels like you should just curl into a ball on the couch, but in the long run, getting up and exercising that wonderful body of yours, no matter how intense, can and will have several benefits both for you and your baby:

- Reduces back pain
- Eases constipation
- May decrease your risk of gestational diabetes, preeclampsia, and cesarean delivery
- Promotes healthy weight gain during pregnancy
- Improves your overall fitness and strengthens your heart and blood vessels
- Helps you to lose the baby weight after your baby is born

The Centers for Disease Control and Prevention recommend that pregnant women get at least 150 minutes of moderate-intensity aerobic activity every week. An aerobic activity is one in which you move large muscles of the body (like those in the legs and arms) in a rhythmic way. Moderate intensity means you are moving enough to raise your heart rate and start sweating. You can still talk normally, but you cannot sing.

Examples of moderate-intensity aerobic activity include brisk walking and general gardening (raking, weeding, or digging). Stop exercising and call your obstetrician or another member of your health care team if you have any of these signs or symptoms:

- Bleeding from the vagina
- Feeling dizzy or faint
- Shortness of breath before starting an exercise
- Headache
- Chest pain
- Calf pain or swelling
- Regular, painful contractions of the uterus
- Fluid leaking from the vagina

Exercises to Avoid During Pregnancy

Don't overdo it! If you want to distill this section down into a simple sentence, that would be it. Some types of exercise involve positions and movements that may be uncomfortable or harmful. While pregnant, do not do any activity that puts you at increased risk of injury, such as the following:

- Contact sports and sports that put you at risk of getting hit in the abdomen, including ice hockey, boxing, soccer, and basketball
- Skydiving

- Activities that may result in a fall, such as downhill snow skiing, water skiing, surfing, off-road cycling, gymnastics, and horseback riding
- Hot yoga or hot Pilates, which may cause you to be overheated
- Scuba diving
- Activities performed above 6,000 feet (if you do not already live at a high altitude)

Pregnant women who exercise regularly have lower risks of gestational diabetes and excess weight gain. They also have fewer aches, more energy, and better muscle tone. Always listen to your body. If you get tired or winded, stop exercising.

Exercises to Try During Pregnancy

4-Point Kneeling: strengthens and tones the abdominal muscles.

- Kneel on all fours. Make sure that your hips are positioned directly over your knees and your shoulders are positioned directly over your hands. Your back should be straight, not curved upward or downward.
- Inhale deeply, and then exhale. As you exhale, pull your abdominal muscles in. Imagine that you are pulling your belly button inward toward your spine. Breathe normally; do not hold your breath. Make sure your back stays straight. This is called "engaging" your abdominal muscles.
- Return to the starting position and repeat five times.

Seated Ball Balance: strengthens abdominal muscles; helps with balance and stability.

- Sit on the center of the ball, keeping your spine in a neutral position. Your feet should be flat on the floor, about hips-width apart.
- Engage your abdominal muscles by imagining that you are pulling your belly button inward toward your spine. Your tailbone (coccyx) should relax. Do not hold your breath. Your arms should be relaxed.
- Raise the left foot off the ground by extending your knee. At the same time, raise your right arm. Hold for five seconds.
- Return to the starting position. Alternate four to six times.

Seated Side Stretch: eases tension on the side of your body; stretches your hip and lateral trunk muscles. May help mitigate stretching/tearing of the transverse abdominis muscle.

- Sit up tall on the center of the ball, keeping your spine in a neutral position and your abdominals engaged. Your feet should be flat on the floor, about hips-width apart. Put your left hand on your right knee.
- Raise your right arm and bend it toward your left side until you feel a gentle stretch. Breathe normally. Do not hunch down or round your shoulders. Hold the stretch for at least five minutes.
- Return to the starting position. Repeat on the other side.

Ball Shoulder Stretch: stretches the upper back, arms, and shoulders.

- Kneel on the floor with the stability ball in front of you.
- Put your hand on either side of the ball.
- Move your buttocks back toward your hips while rolling the ball in front of you. Keep your eyes on the floor; do not arch your neck. Go only as far as is comfortable for you to feel a gentle stretch. Hold the stretch for a few seconds.
- Return to the starting position. Repeat four to six times.

Ball Wall Squat: strengthens muscles in the legs and buttocks.

- Place the exercise ball against a wall. Stand and firmly press the ball into the wall using your low back.
- Distribute your weight between both feet. With a slow, controlled movement, squat down while firmly pressing against the ball. Do not let your knees collapse inward. Keep your feet flat, and avoid lifting your heels. Maintain an open chest and avoid rounding your shoulders.
- Start with squatting halfway if you cannot squat all the way down. Caution: If you have any knee pain, do not do this exercise.
- Repeat four to six times, working up to 10-12 times.

Kneeling Heel Touch: tones muscles of the upper and lower back; tones abdominals; stretches arm muscles.

- Kneel on an exercise mat.
- Using a slow, controlled movement, rotate your torso to the right. Bring your right hand back and touch your left heel. Extend your left arm above your head for balance.
- Exhale when you reach back. Rotate the trunk to look back at your foot to increase the rotation. Avoid tensing your buttocks or hunching your shoulders, which will hinder your movement.
- Return to the starting position. Alternate four to six times.

Feel Prepared?

Pregnancy is a beautiful experience, however, it can get marred by several complications, including pelvic floor disorders. As such, we should aspire to make the most of the experience, and that's why we should take several precautions, especially before getting pregnant. With pre-pregnancy planning, in addition to visiting a gynecologist to get an overall body check done, also have a further check-up with a women's health PT to have your pelvic muscles checked thoroughly so that we can take the necessary corrective measures if necessary. We will also check your back, neck, ribcage, etc, as you're a whole person and the entire body goes through changes during this special time in your life.

Also, during pregnancy issues can arise. Consequently, it is essential to keep all appointments and report anything that seems out of the ordinary, no matter how insignificant it may seem. Doing this can help prevent further complications and even miscarriages. Being a good caretaker of your pelvic floor is just the beginning. It is the building block that you can use to encourage general well-being at the beginning, middle, and end of your pregnancy. As we will see more throughout this book, there is no "big fix." There is only the want and will to improve your life and health so that you can be the best mama you can possibly be.

Go ahead, Mama, take a breath and soften.

WHAT CAN GO WRONG WHEN IT GOES RIGHT: MISCARRIAGE

I t is not my intention to sugar-coat any moment of your, or my, journey. You are strong and the realities of early pregnancy often include a word so many of us wish to avoid—miscarriage. My own story begins with such a word, but it does not end with it. The more we can share about this oft-overlooked stage without stigma or fear, the better we can understand how to care for ourselves after. Take a deep breath and join me as we step into the hard parts together and come out the other side, hand-in-hand.

A Culture of Silence

My husband and I felt broken and devastated after we realized that we were losing my pregnancy. Two weeks went by and I had a visit with my doctor at what should have been my OB workup visit. When I checked in with the front desk, a woman handed me a cup for a urine sample. I handed it back to her and let her know I had just had a miscarriage. She apologized and sent me back to the private patient's room. The sad smile on her face was one I knew I had given clients before. The doctor came in and expressed her sympathies and asked a few questions. I found it strange that she didn't insist on an ultrasound to verify the miscarriage. She did have me get blood work done to check my HCG levels, which we later found out were extremely high despite the fact that HCG usually decreases once a pregnancy is lost.

My doctor was already trying to advise me on procedures, such as dilation and curettage, while I continued to bleed and mourn what could have been. My ever-supportive husband was not convinced. He did his own research and was convinced from day one that I could possibly be carrying twins. We decided to book an ultrasound before moving forward on my OB's advice for our peace of mind.

The day of the ultrasound I was a ball of nerves. I even arrived five minutes late, which was seriously uncharacteristic of me. The ultrasound technician was friendly enough, but I was perturbed to hear her ask if I was excited for the ultrasound with that sing-songy tone that under usual conditions may have brought a smile to my face. She must have not looked over my chart very carefully. I informed her that I had had a miscarriage and that we just wanted to check if I had to have a procedure to remove tissue next, something that I didn't even want to think about.

Her face changed from casual pleasantness to confusion. She looked from me to the black and gray screen. Then, back to me.

"Are you sure? What makes you think you had a miscarriage?"

I told her that I had seen the fetal sac in the toilet with copious amounts of blood. It was pretty hard to miss. The technician told me to take a look at the screen. I did, my body vibrating with nerves and anxiety. It felt like hours for my eyes to adjust and for my brain to comprehend the blobby mass of movement that followed the wand's adjustment. There it was. I saw the cutest little half-inch baby moving around.

I was in disbelief and asked the technician several times to check and recheck for a heartbeat. She said it was there, beating loud and clear. I was so stirred up, I could feel my eyes swelling with tears starting to roll down my cheeks. Tears of joy and sadness.

I had been carrying twins. I did, indeed, miscarry a fetus, but only one of the two that my body nourished. After researching, this is not as uncommon as one may believe. The many reasons for a pregnancy to self-terminate during early stages remain statistically relevant in the case of multiples. In my case, a single twin was unable to continue past that early stage of development while my son was. I have never felt a more poignant moment of bitter-sweet. My loss was still a loss, but hope continued to grow.

I was 8.5 weeks at this time and decided to look for a new doctor that would see me through my entire pregnancy and delivery after our experience. I couldn't help but still go over in my head various questions that crossed my mind about the miscarriage and remaining pregnancy. They stayed with me as did the fear and the grief, but there was joy there, too.

Before it happened to me, I had no idea how many women suffer from miscarriage. I did not know that a good percentage of the women in my life had experienced this secret loss. As I shared my story, more and more followed. A shared pain and a sisterhood grew between us and I realized I am not alone and neither are they.

What Went Wrong?

Miscarriage is the most prevalent complication of pregnancy. Between 15-20% of all clinically recognized pregnancies end in miscarriages.[22] A miscarriage can occur before the 12th week of pregnancy. Pregnant women miscarry due to an abnormality in the chromosomes formed or problems with the fetus's development. It may be a result of:

- Infections
- Radiation, toxic substance in the environment or the home
- Abnormal hormonal levels
- Stress
- Extreme cases of diabetes
- Effects of some prescription drugs, like Accutane
- Uterine abnormalities
- Issues with the cervix
- Lifestyles
- Substance abuse

What Symptoms May Signal a Miscarriage?

Heavier bleeding than usual, spotting, cramping, abdominal bleeding, back pains, pelvic pain, fluid from the vagina, nausea, diarrhea, tissue coming from the vagina, disappearance of other pregnancy symptoms, and unexplained weakness can indicate a miscarriage.

Why Do People Shy Away From Discussing Miscarriage If it is Common?

Cultural and societal norms place a lot of pressure on issues surrounding childbirth and pregnancy loss. Some people go to the extent of concealing their pregnancies before the 14th week because the baby's chances of surviving are small. Discussions about miscarriage are often considered a social taboo, meaning that very few people openly talk about it for fear of offending someone.

According to research, about one in every five pregnancies ends in a miscarriage[23], making this phenomenon relatively common. However, family, close friends, and sometimes partners of women who've miscarried don't understand their grief, which can have long-term implications on their mental health and well-being.

What Are Some Possible Physical and Emotional Effects of Miscarriage?

If you had a miscarriage, you would need some time for your body to recover. Some common physical and emotional effects include:

- Vaginal bleeding (spotting or light bleeding) for up to a week
- Lower abdominal pain
- Cramping for one to two days
- Breast discomfort and milk leakage for up to a week
- Sense of isolation
- Profound grief, stress, and anxiety
- Symptoms of depression

Are All Cases of Miscarriage Like What I Experienced?

No, women may experience different types of miscarriages.

- When a woman experiences bleeding and cramping with an open cervix, it is inevitable that she has miscarried a pregnancy.
- Some may lose a pregnancy when they bleed with little or no pain and a closed cervix, but most pregnancies may survive.
- Some also experience an incomplete miscarriage. This miscarriage occurs when the body does not expel all the tissues from

the pregnancy. In a complete miscarriage, the body removes all the tissues from the pregnancy.

- Lastly, some might experience a missed miscarriage, where the fetus dies or fails to develop, but is not discharged by the body.

Was It My Fault?

It was no fault of yours just as my miscarriage was no fault of mine. Typically, one cannot prevent cases of miscarriages caused by chromosomal abnormalities or other problems with the fetus. Age and a history of miscarriages are a factor in some women, but not necessarily a high risk factor on their own. The only instances where a pregnant woman can do something substantial to prevent a miscarriage is when women who smoke, do drugs, or drink stop when pregnant. These are habits that increase the probability of losing a pregnancy. Needless to say, a healthy lifestyle helps to ensure a healthy baby.

Can I Get Pregnant Again After a Miscarriage?

Definitely! Most women can get pregnant shortly after they miscarry. Some even have multiple miscarriages before giving birth.

Coping with miscarriage differs between different people. Some take it as a blip and move on, while others don't. Grieving is okay, no matter how you choose to do so. You and your partner should always allow yourself time to process what has happened—the joy that the pregnancy once brought as well as the sadness. Most of all, always be kind to yourself and remember that in the end, life must go on.

Go ahead, Mama, take a breath and soften.

PREGNANCY: A STUDY IN HOPE AND NEW BEGINNINGS

My Pregnancy Journey

Where to begin…I was still pregnant with my son when I started writing this book. If I am being honest, it felt bizarre to be speaking these words and revealing this information to you, someone who I do not know, yet have this bond with as a woman. We are connected in a certain way even though we are still separated in so many other ways. Now you know things about me that I keep close to the chest in so many other situations.

It wasn't necessarily easy. To me, it seemed like it was always the lucky ladies who happened to conceive whenever they wanted to, while I had to spend many years hoping and waiting for it to happen. That mindset hurts. It caused pain and anxiety in me. When I became pregnant, I realized that was not even my greatest test. Instead, it was the secrecy around, not my longing, but my loss.

Why is no one talking about miscarriages? I suspect this is a major reason I wanted to tell my experience in the first place: to let women know that the process of conceiving and being pregnant is a roller coaster ride and that you're not alone. Despite reports that 20% of women suffer miscarriages,[24] you still believe that you are the only one enduring this. Even now, having my baby in my arms, it nags at me. It is hard to believe that so much time has passed since those two lines appeared and those tears that fell shortly after.

I was quite depressed and miserable during the first trimester. I stopped caring about things I used to enjoy. I was completely disinterested in anything. It seemed better to talk about it than keep it to myself. After speaking with my doctor, I was relieved to learn that my symptoms were not caused by a serious medical issue, but by hormonal changes. I was told that the problem would be resolved in a matter of weeks. And, it did.

Getting encouragement like this from a doctor versus getting lectured by a friend for "not being happy about being pregnant" was groundbreaking for me. Without judgment surrounding me, I could see clearly, I could sense hope and come to understand myself. It did teach me something about judgment, however. It is never a good idea to rush to that place where you may inflict pain on a fellow sister simply because you lack understanding.

That is what we are here to do. To understand. Women, for as long as we have been helping each other through pregnancy and birth, have known that the best way to come to a mutual understanding is to share our experiences. To relate on that most basic level. This is why I wish to share with you my personal experience with my pregnancy so that maybe, just maybe, you will see a bit of your own journey in me and find comfort.

Let's start with the symptoms. I had a poor mood due to hormonal changes (I only felt it for the first 10 weeks) and reluctance to eat (I felt so nauseous!). I developed a heightened sense of smell and aversions to things like coffee or my husband's cologne and often felt utterly exhausted and hence would need frequent naps to complete a workday. Breaking off to go to the bathroom all. the. time. was not fun in the least. On top of that, despite my small intake of tea, I felt like I had overeaten.

It was not all for naught. Seeing our developing baby during our ultrasound scans highlights my pregnancy, while bye-bye nausea around week 8 is a relief. We were also feeling better mentally, with the difficult weeks behind us. My pregnancy was progressing easily and naturally and I told family and friends the exciting news.

During the first trimester, I found some things essential for my survival. Ginger tea and toast kept me from starving and sick bags allowed me to possibly get sick at work with absolute grace. The ability to nap also helped. You know, to not want to lay down and die instead.

The second trimester was better. In fact, it was great! I had a massive surge of energy and delight. Every day, day in and day out. No more naps for me and those sick bags, forget about it. During the last few weeks of the second trimester, I did experience a small soreness in my pelvic region. When it disappeared, it was a huge relief. I have known quite a few ladies who were struck hard by it, and I was fortunate to avoid it completely. Furthermore, it was great to appreciate the pleasure of eating and scents once again. Haha! Of course, I had heard from everyone how fantastic this pregnancy time is. Even amid a pandemic. It's a relief that the trimester went so well.

This was also when I got some adorable bloating and could finally see my expanding belly. A lot of excitement! There was some round ligament pain (since everything is stretching). Also, some pelvic and lower back pain. But that was okay because I was enjoying my favorite meal again and familiar scents. I had my morning routine down, which started with a 30-minute bike ride on my NordicTrack. This not only helped get me going for the day, it really shaped my mindset and put me in a good mental perspective for the day ahead. The bulk of my energy was in the morning and I found when I got my exercising done early, I made better choices throughout the day.

I felt all of the initial flutters, and then baby kicks and wiggles around the beginning of this trimester. I was very excited to see my growing bulge. The anatomy scan was amazing. Lastly, we discovered the gender of our child, ensuring a well-stocked nursery and having everything necessary in place! We were so excited to welcome a baby boy into the world!

The third trimester was a real mixture for me. The challenges only really began in the vicinity of 32 weeks. It was on tenterhooks. Just a reminder for anyone who does not already know, if you happen to see a woman in her 3rd trimester, do not urge her to "get some sleep while she can." If you do, you are the worst. To begin with, you can't hoard sleep.

You won't sleep straight through the night during your third trimester and that is okay. That happens notably after 32 weeks. If you have trouble sleeping at night, taking naps during the day is the solution. We also had two sonograms to check the growth of the fetus. I grew one week beyond my standard measurement at 28 weeks, and I also progressed a week further by the time I was 31 weeks pregnant.

I'll note that after my first ultrasound, the doctor's made slight comments and suggestions that I may have to be induced early due to the baby's size, length not weight, and my age, as I had recently turned 35 and apparently that puts me at "advanced maternal age." At the time of that ultrasound, I was only 18 weeks, which is extremely early in pregnancy to put any stock in knowing exactly how big the baby will be. That is where I tended to get frustrated, by the little comments I kept hearing from the doctors, like, "Don't try and be a hero, interventions are good." Like, way to defeat my spirits before I've even gone into labor!

Thankfully, the doula we hired was excellent and reassured us every step of the way that natural birth was 100% possible and achievable. We decided together to give birth in the alternative birthing center with the help of the midwife on call who would be in constant communication with the OB on call. Our li'l guy was in great hands.

Well, there it is. How my pregnancy went right up to the tricky labor and delivery part, which you'll get a taste of a bit later. Your pregnancy may look like mine or it may not, but that's why I share. It is overwhelming looking at it all in one place, right? It's okay if you are, I was too when my friends and family shared their own stories. Take a little at a time and do what you can to prepare. Most of all though, never lose sight of why you are doing it.

Go ahead, Mama, take a breath and soften.

HOW TO DEAL WITH SPD IN PREGNANCY (WHEN YOUR PELVIS IS LITERALLY TEARING ITSELF APART)

What to Know About Symphysis Pubis Dysfunction & How to Manage It

There are plenty of symptoms that we know come with pregnancy, and it can be a bit overwhelming if it is your first pregnancy and you aren't sure what to expect. The important thing to remember is that each woman is different, and no two pregnancies are the exact same. Symphysis pubis dysfunction (SPD), aka lightning crotch, is just as uncomfortable as it sounds.

SPD is a condition that primarily occurs during pregnancy and it is characterized by discomfort in the pelvic region. With symphysis pubis dysfunction, the pelvis becomes very stiff and possibly uneven during this time, and the severity of the discomfort varies among each individual. Another name for this condition is pelvic girdle pain, and today we are going to discuss everything you may be wondering about when it comes to it as well as some helpful tips if you are showcasing symptoms of this and would like some much-needed relief.

What is the Symphysis Pubis and Where is it Located?

The symphysis pubis is the joint where the pubic bones join together via cartilage, and it is located in the front region of the pelvis and near the perineum. The symphysis pubis ensures that you are able to move comfortably while maintaining pelvic health by keeping it secure and in place. The body, of course, goes through many changes during pregnancy, especially in the pelvic region. When it comes to symphysis pubis dysfunction, the pelvic ligaments may relax and the cartilage that comprises this joint softens due to the various hormonal changes that come into play during pregnancy. Combined with the baby's weight that is adding pressure to the pubic symphysis region, this softening translates into anything from mild discomfort to severe pain in the pelvic floor, back, and thighs while participating in certain activities.

When symphysis pubis dysfunction takes place, the pelvic bones that are being held together by this joint may become uneven, which is a major contributing factor of the pain that is experienced with this condition. Symphysis pubis dysfunction does not occur in every pregnancy, and it can happen in other instances too—albeit this is not as common. There is not too much research regarding subsequent pregnancies when you have experienced pelvic girdle pain before, but the treatment options that we are going to talk about shortly can help exponentially when it comes to lessening the discomfort that SPD creates.

Who Does This Affect?

While symphysis pubis dysfunction can affect individuals that are not pregnant, it is most often associated with pregnancy. Some research shows that around 1 in every 5 pregnant women may experience varying degrees of symphysis pubis dysfunction.[25] This condition onsets during the 2nd or 3rd trimesters more often than the 1st, although it can really begin at any time during pregnancy. The good news is that SPD and the pain that is associated with it typically vanishes within a week after birth, and if it is taking longer than that there are many treatment options out there that are available to help you remediate this issue.

If you are concerned that SPD will make for a more painful or difficult delivery, this is not necessarily the case. There is some evidence[25] that even shows that SPD might make the process of labor and delivery easier, since the pelvis is more relaxed, softer, and mobile than usual. Symphysis pubis dysfunction often makes it harder to open the legs wide, which is necessary for a vaginal birth, so it is vital to work in the following treatment options to reduce any pain as much as possible leading up to birth.

Factors that may increase the risk of SPD[26] include: being overweight or obese during pregnancy, having an injury to the pelvis, having a history of low back pain, or experiencing pelvic pain in a previous pregnancy. Another factor includes one hip that is chronically bothering you or tight. Once pregnancy hormones kick in and your pelvis and your symphysis pubis become more flexible, this can create malalignment.

Treatment Options

There are a few different treatment options when it comes to this condition, but the first course of action is typically physical therapy. Physical therapy has shown to be highly effective for increasing the stability and function of your pelvic bones and muscles, and this form of treatment is wonderful for reducing the pain that is experienced with SPD. Hydrotherapy is another great option for pregnant women that have SPD, as this diminishes any added stress from your joints, is highly relaxing, and maintains stability.

If you are seeing a women's health physical therapist for SPD, they will likely provide you with several different exercises that you can do regularly on your own time to improve your symptoms with it in addition to manual therapy. Hands-on body work with a specialist's eyes on your body can help reveal any compensation patterns and manually release restrictions in ways that cannot be done at home.[27] Some exercises include strengthening, for example: side-lying leg raises, seated Kegels, lumbar rotation stretches, seated clamshells, lateral walks. TENS therapy,[25] or transcutaneous electrical nerve stimulation unit, might be recommended if there is not a great response to physical therapy. TENS therapy involves sending minor electrical stimulation to a specific area in order to relieve the pain—in this case the pelvis region. Another thing to note is it's important to keep your legs together when you're sleeping. I suggest stacking your knees and putting a pillow between them if you need to. Acupuncture can be beneficial during this time, and pharmaceutical treatment is typically a last resort option, but there are some options that are safe to take while pregnant if all else fails.

There are also special supportive belts that are made particularly for those that are struggling with SPD pain, and these work by alleviating the persistent pressure on the pelvis. In very severe cases that are not as common, crutches or a wheelchair might be suggested if no other forms of treatment are working.

Activity Modification

Symphysis pubis dysfunction may cause issues when it comes to mobility due to the pain and unevenness of the pubic region, so it may be necessary to modify some of your activities so that there is the least amount of pain possible. Some activity modifications that have shown to help significantly include:

1. Take Smaller Steps
   Walking may become more uncomfortable than usual when you are experiencing symphysis pubis dysfunction since the pelvis can become uneven with this condition, but taking smaller steps than normal can reduce the pain considerably since the discomfort can onset more when the pelvis is stretching more.

2. Sleep on Your Side
   Sleeping on your side and with a pillow between your legs has proven to be the most comfortable way to sleep when SPD has been diagnosed. This sleeping position reduces the weight that is placed on the pelvis and will ensure that you get the most restful night's sleep possible.

3. Walk Up Stairs Sideways
   Just as walking with big steps can create more pain with SPD, stairs are not your friend if you are dealing with this condition. Taking stairs sideways is the best course of action, as this method certifies that you are putting the least amount of strain on your pelvis compared to walking up them regularly. Avoid symmetrical movements like lunges.

4. Use a Seat Cushion

Simple things like sitting can become extremely uncomfortable with SPD, so it is a great idea to purchase a seat or lumbar cushion to use so that you can relax with ease and the utmost comfort.

5. Keep Knees Close Together
   Similarly, with taking smaller steps while you walk, you will want to keep your knees as close together as you can whenever possible. This will come in handy when you're doing something like getting out of bed in the morning or when you're shifting directions. This will reduce the tension on your pelvic floor and keep you much more comfortable.

While symphysis pubis dysfunction is common in pregnancy, a lot of women find it manageable and heal from it quickly after labor. SPD does not affect your chances of being able to have a vaginal birth if that is a concern of yours, and there are, thankfully, plenty of treatment options available to anyone that is dealing with this condition. As long as you work in a form of therapy as well as activity modifications during pregnancy and after labor, SPD is something that is typically managed very successfully.

Yoga and Pilates can also be helpful, but it's important to know there are certain movements that can exacerbate things. In many cases, I advise avoiding any deep squats or lunges. Legs wide and uneven will exacerbate your pain. Legs close together and parallel is optimal.

Pelvic floor pain should be taken seriously before it gets worse. Know that: you are not complaining; you are not a weak link.

CARPAL TUNNEL SYNDROME DURING PREGNANCY

verything hurts. I remember groaning this to myself more than once during my pregnancy and I am sure you are, too. From my fingers to my toes, discomfort began to set in during the later months of my pregnancy. If this is you too, you may be suffering from a potential side effect called carpal tunnel syndrome (CTS).

Thankfully, my case was resolved right after I gave birth, but it was quite challenging for me at times, especially when at work given the nature of what my work entails. It helped that I have successfully treated many patients with carpal tunnel syndrome over the years and now had the chance to experience it first hand (pun intended). For you, let's start at the basics.

What is Carpal Tunnel Syndrome?

Carpal tunnel syndrome refers to a condition resulting from the swelling that occurs around the nerves within the wrist. The carpal tunnel is a narrow corridor surrounded by bones and ligaments. It also houses tendons and the median nerve, which is the main nerve of the front of the forearm and travels through the base of your hand. If you develop this condition, it means the carpal tunnel has become swollen and is now placing pressure against your very sensitive median nerve. This is the reason for the pain, numbness, and tingling you experience in one or both wrists. CTS is particularly common among pregnant women, with about 3 to 5 of every 10 women developing this condition during pregnancy.[28,29]

During pregnancy, you experience hormonal fluctuations, which may lead to fluid accumulation, causing swelling. It is this swelling that then results in nerve hypersensitivity by pushing against the median nerve in your carpal tunnel. The sometimes constantly increasing pressure within the carpal tunnel incites pain in your hands and wrists.[30]

Though rare, you may notice symptoms of CTS during your second trimester, but the condition is more pronounced in the third trimester. In some instances, women have developed this condition after birth. In another research,[31] published in 2014, the investigators identified other factors that place pregnant women at risk of developing carpal tunnel syndrome, such as gestational hypertension, gestational diabetes, obesity, excessive gestational weight gain, and consistent work involving the use of your hands and wrists.

How Do I Relieve My Symptoms?

There are several at-home remedies and medical treatments that you can safely use to get relief from carpal tunnel syndrome. However, the appropriate treatment is dependent on varying factors, such as the stage you are in your pregnancy and the severity of your symptoms.

If you work from a desk, practice developing a good posture for your wrists and arms as a whole. Also, practice taking a break every 20 minutes or as often as possible. Rest your hands by elevating them, possibly on pillows, when they are not being used throughout the day and even while you sleep, or use ice wrapped in a towel to place on your wrist for about 10-minute intervals. Do this multiple times throughout the day, as it will help to reduce the swelling.[32] Most simply, limit your engagement in activities that require you to bend your wrist. I also recommend my patients to try practicing yoga, as study shows[32] that it may reduce pain and increase grip strength.

If you have access to medical providers who can provide assistance, they have several resources to offer. They may try applying a splint to keep your wrist in a neutral position or help you stretch the front of the neck as well as the upper trapezius group and levator scapulae muscles. Physical therapy can also help to relieve pain and increase function in your wrist and arm.

Can I Prevent Carpal Tunnel from Developing?

If you are concerned about developing carpal tunnel syndrome during pregnancy, there are a few steps you can take to prevent the condition. They are quite similar to the home remedies for treating the actual condition. You can reduce the time you spend doing tasks, such as typing, sewing, or knitting. If you do continue with these activities, take breaks to move your hands around and stretch. For those of us who spend time on our phones, avoid scrolling on your phone for extended periods. Basically, take care of your hands and wrists as best you can.

Will Having Carpal Tunnel Syndrome During Pregnancy Affect My Pregnancy or Baby?

Carpal tunnel syndrome during pregnancy will not directly affect your baby or your pregnancy. However, because it impedes the mobility of your hands it may indirectly affect both baby and pregnancy if you are unable to do your everyday tasks. Additionally, there are other conditions that could be the cause of your CTS, such as preeclampsia (high blood pressure that develops during pregnancy). This condition can become life-threatening to you and your baby, as such, if you develop sudden severe swelling it is an indication that something is wrong.

Typically, carpal tunnel syndrome resolves itself after you have given birth. It subsides because the excess fluid that caused swelling and pressure leaves your body. This may take weeks or months, as it is dependent on how quickly your body recovers after delivery.

Bear in mind that you should at least be seeing a reduction in symptoms within the first 12 months after having your baby, so if you are still experiencing symptoms, speak with your doctor.

I recommend early intervention from your doctor because of its association with the development of preeclampsia, which is hypertension marked by high protein in the urine. Because this condition is so dangerous, you must speak with your doctor right away if you notice sudden, severe swelling in your face, hands, ankles, and feet. You may also experience vision changes, nausea, vomiting, headaches, and difficulty breathing.

If you do not receive prompt and appropriate treatment for preeclampsia, it can result in critical complications, such as premature birth, intrauterine growth restriction (when the fetus does not grow as expected), and placental abruption (occurs when the placenta separates from the uterus). Even if you do not have that generalized and excessive swelling, once you develop carpal tunnel syndrome symptoms, speak to your doctor. Remember, CTS can cause significant nerve damage, so don't delay.

Ladies, pregnancy is beautiful and although marred with certain challenges, you can still experience bliss. Therefore to avoid being weighed down with issues like CTS, try to seek medical attention as soon as you notice changes in your body. Listen to your therapists and doctor's advice and rest those arms and wrists as much as possible and don't forget to stretch your neck as the nerves that come out of your neck also go down to your hands. It's imperative to treat the symptoms, but look elsewhere for the root cause.

Go ahead, Mama, take a breath and soften.

LABOR AND BIRTH

The big moment has come and it is time to finally meet your new baby. Today is the day that you step into that new and exciting phase of life: motherhood. Don't worry, I was scared too. Whether it is your first time feeling those tell-tale contractions or your tenth, the second you realize that this is it there is no mistaking the adrenaline rush that comes with early labor. Hopefully, you have a supportive birthing partner there to hold your hand and a medical team ready for anything. There is only one goal here and that is to meet your bundle of joy in the healthiest way possible.

If you have ever been a group of women when birth stories come up, you know that it is different. You may have quick labor and barely make it to the hospital parking lot. You may be induced and end up laboring for days. C-section, vaginal, no one is entirely sure how your experience will go. That is why I won't try and cover every single aspect of the process and instead tell you about my own experience, from my birth plan to the birth of my son, Teddy. I also would like to encourage you to reach out to the other women in your life. We are a sisterhood and this is really where the lifelong support begins.

WHY DO WOMEN GIVE BIRTH ON THEIR BACKS?

Research has shown that, historically, women used to give birth in an upright position either by sitting, squatting, or kneeling. There is even evidence of them using assistive devices, such as stools to support themselves during the process. However, traditional standards have now "dictated" that labor and delivery be carried out in the supine or back-lying position. The typical healthcare facilities insist on using this position, even though there is much evidence to suggest that other positions are more beneficial and conducive to birthing. So, we wonder why women started giving birth on their backs? Let's have a look together.

The Historical Concept

Many believe that the primary reason women began to deliver on their backs was for the convenience of men who wanted to witness the process.

The idea of the "males view" is said to have arisen from the desire of King Louis XIV from 17th-century France who enjoyed his wives giving birth in a back-lying position. This theory is even explored in a <u>study</u> titled, "The Evolution of Maternal Birthing Position."[33]

The author explains that the king liked watching the birthing process, however, his view was often blocked when the birth took place on a birthing stool. This obstruction annoyed him greatly, so he decided to introduce a new reclining position. Since then, the practice of back-down delivery caught on and became standard practice.[33]

Socioeconomic Status

Is it really believed that women who squat during delivery are of lower socioeconomic status? Some people believe that socioeconomic status played a major role in determining what positions are used during delivery because squatting was seen as a lower-class position. It could be associated with the trend started by King Louis XIV, but we can't say for sure, as we were unable to find evidence of these claims. However, we did come across information showing that education and experience may affect the way women choose birthing positions. This study[34] indicated that highly educated and older women were more likely to use non-supine birthing[35] positions, which to a degree suggests inequalities in position choice.

Medical Expertise and Convenience

The experts believe that maternal birthing positions are influenced by women's empowerment, age, parity, culture, the healthcare attendants who are primary caregivers during the labor process, among other factors. In one study[36] that included both medical professionals and new mothers, it was evidenced that the birthing position used by the women during delivery was, of course, the supine position.

The study[33] also revealed that this position was chosen and agreed to because of the midwives' knowledge and professional experience. It had nothing to do with the women's choice. In that same study, the authors highlighted that the healthcare professionals prefer to use the supine position, for a matter of convenience for them. That is, it facilitated the easy monitoring of the woman and her unborn baby during labor and delivery.

Modern Reasons

While the back-lying position was introduced for a matter of convenience and status, there are several other reasons today why it is continuously used as the standard birthing position. These reasons are discussed at length in these articles:[37,38]

- Technological advances- increased efficiency in the placement and use of epidural anesthesia for enhanced pain control, fetal monitoring, and anesthesia.
- Health condition- with certain medical conditions, women are encouraged to use the supine position. For example, with high-risk pregnancies where the baby and mother require constant monitoring.
- Forceps or a ventouse (vacuum)- if during birth a mother needs to get assistance to help the baby out, she will need to lie on her back.

MINIMIZING VAGINAL TEARING DURING BIRTH

ringing a life into this world is such a blessing. But, a blessing is not necessarily something filled with butterflies and rainbows. Sometimes, the most beautiful thing in the world involves the moment many of us dread from the second we realize it can happen. The vaginal tear, whether you experience it or not, is usually not far from your mind when giving birth.

The process or journey to birth itself can be tedious. The pregnancy and delivery experience may vary among mothers, as some will have a beautiful, stress-free journey, while others may have risks and complications. A vaginal tear, which is called a perineal laceration, is an injury incurred on the area that separates your vagina and rectum—the perineum—and it is one of the most common complications of labor and birth.

Vaginal tearing happens quite often. In fact, according to the Royal College of Obstetricians and Gynecologists,[39] approximately 9 in every 10 first-time mothers who have a vaginal birth will experience some sort of tear. Luckily, there are some ways expectant mothers can try to mitigate vaginal tears during delivery, and in this chapter, we look at a few ways that can be done. We will also explore why women give birth on their backs and whether we should massage or not massage the perineum before labor.

It's always helpful to know which positions your provider supports so you can be sure that everyone is on the same page. I recommend changing positions every 30 minutes, which can help the baby move down into the pelvis. Utilizing gravity in an upright pushing position is a great option to best prevent tearing of the vaginal tissue, also called a perineal laceration.

5 Best Birthing Positions to Minimize Vaginal Tearing During Birth

Vaginal tears can occur for several reasons, including:

- First vaginal birth
- Episiotomy
- The baby is big (weighs over 4kg/ 9lb)
- You have to push for an extended period
- You have an instrumental-assisted vaginal delivery where forceps or another device were used

Positioning during delivery can help to combat some of these issues and there are several positions that you can choose to use when delivering your baby. However, some of these positions are more beneficial than others. While some positions utilize the assistance of gravity to provide a much smoother and less stressful birthing process, others don't. Research[40] suggests that women should avoid giving birth on their back and should follow their body's urge to push. So, let's take a look at those positions that take advantage of gravity to assist with reducing vaginal tearing.

1. Squatting

In this position, the foot of your bed would be lowered and the birthing bar attached so that you can lean forward in a squat while resting your head and arms on top of the bar. Squatting is one of those positions that take advantage of gravity to help your baby move down into your pelvis. In addition, squatting increases the size of the pelvis, which means more space for your baby to pass through easier. Additionally, when you squat during labor it strengthens the feeling of thrust and relaxation of your perineal muscles.

These benefits mean that you are required to push less forcefully during delivery, and as such, less assistance, like an episiotomy or forceps, is needed. A study published in 2007 by the National Library of Medicine,[41] looked at 200 women who had recently given birth. One set of moms used the squatting position, while the other set remained in the traditional position. The study[41] findings suggest that the squatting position may result in less instrumental deliveries, the extension of episiotomies, and vaginal tears.

Cons:

Although quite beneficial, squatting is the most exhausting position. Consequently, it is generally used in combination with side-lying, semi-sitting, and kneeling. You will also rest between contractions and that is highly encouraged.

2. Sitting Upright

To sit upright while giving birth, you will lean forward slightly in a semi-squat. Your hands are placed on each knee with your legs opened, and during each push, you will extend your elbows outwards. In this upright delivery position, you are using the natural gravitational pull to aid with the process. Sitting upright expedites the delivery by helping the baby to move downward and out more easily.

When you sit upright during delivery, the gravitational pull reduces the effort you need to push and so, instead of going against gravity, you are working with it. Therefore, it shortens the delivery time for you, which in turn reduces the amount of stress placed on your perineum, making it less susceptible to tearing.

According to a piece of research,[42] published in 2014 by the National Center for Biotechnology Information, the sitting position takes advantage of gravity, the use of lumbar massage, and facilitates an increased pelvic diameter with better fetal alignment to the pelvis. These features were then found to reduce the need for an epidural or an assisted birth with various devices.[42] Plus, this position is ideal for resting.

Cons:
The sitting upright position may increase the pressure on the sacrum, adding the risk of trauma. Additionally, it is not recommended for women with hypertension.

3. Lying Sideways

To assume the side-lying position, you will need to lie on one side, with the legs opened, pulled toward the chest, and knees bent during contractions to support pushing. This position tends to make your contractions more effective, as such, you are in labor for a shorter period, which decreases chances of tearing or the need for an episiotomy.

Being extremely tense during delivery is one other factor that can contribute to the need for an episiotomy or the use of an assistive device. The tension you exude can even cause a vaginal tear; however, in the side-lying position, gravity and other benefits, such as increased relaxation and the possibility of resting more between contractions, reduces the likelihood of an episiotomy, tear, or assistive device use, as seen in this study.[43]

Cons:

In the side-lying position, it can be easy to become very passive, causing you not to push hard enough. Also, it may be difficult for you to hold your legs open, as no one is able to support them entirely for you.

4. On All Fours or Kneeling

In this position, you would be kneeling and bent forward while supporting your weight with your arms. This is another gravity-using position that allows you to rest more and use less energy while pushing. You may also have a shorter delivery time because of the action of the gravitational force that helps you to push the baby out. The less resistance you have and the less need for pushing means the less likely you are to get a vaginal tear, as discussed in this scientific article.[37] The article further explains that Irish and New Zealand expert midwives favor the all-fours position for preserving the perineum intact at birth.[37]

Because kneeling helps you to take advantage of gravity and move your baby down into the pelvis with a bit less effort, the contractions can be less painful yet way more productive, causing your baby to be well-aligned in your pelvis. This alignment again helps to reduce delivery time and the amount of pushing you need to do.

Also, according to this study,[44] kneeling on all fours is one of the birthing positions that take the weight off the sacrum, making it more flexible, thus reducing the risk of a perineal tear. Lastly, similar to squatting and standing, the dimensions of the pelvis can be maximized by the hands-and-knees position.

Cons:

In this position, it can sometimes be challenging for the healthcare worker to efficiently assess and assist you with the delivery.

5. Standing

To assume this position, you are simply in an upright position standing by yourself or against a form of support, such as a bed, chair, or partner. Standing in an upright position helps with positioning your pelvis, which causes it to increase the opening by approximately 15% more than the traditional back-lying position.[45] Standing helps you to utilize the natural push from gravity to help the baby move down into the pelvis.

As indicated in a 2019 study review,[45] giving birth in the standing position might facilitate the rotation and descent of your baby's head, therefore resulting in the decrease in duration of the second stage of labor, and by now we know that reducing delivery time means lessening the pressure placed on the perineum. So, that's a reduction in the likelihood of you receiving a vaginal tear. Further, it means you may not need a device or other assistance since you won't have a prolonged birthing process.

In addition to that, when you give birth in the standing position, it takes the weight off the sacrum, decreasing the risk for perineal injuries and the need for an episiotomy, as was reported in this article.[44] Again, while being more productive, with this position, your contractions may feel less painful, as it aids with lengthening your upper body to help your baby become better aligned with the angle of your pelvis.

Cons:

This position can be rather tiring for you and your partner as well, so you will need to take as much rest between contractions as possible.

6. The Traditional Supine or Back-lying Position

Although history reveals that this was not the original and natural birthing position, over the years, lying on the back with legs open rose to become the norm. However, recent studies[37] have suggested that the supine position should be avoided because of its propensity to increase women's risk of severe perineal trauma. This scientific article[37] further explains that in the supine position, women experience comparatively longer labor, greater pain, and more fetal heart rate patterns.

In another research article,[38] the authors pointed out that in all women studied, the comparison between those who used the back-lying position versus those who used the upright position showed a marked reduction in duration of the second stage in the upright group.

The back-lying position may not be ideal for preventing or reducing perineal trauma; however, it does make for greater visibility.

Cons:

The supine position works against gravity, which causes you to use more effort for pushing and can delay the delivery process. Also, it causes your pelvis to become smaller and increases the need for instrument-assisted delivery or an episiotomy.

To Massage the Perineum Before Labor or Not?

To massage or not to massage? This is an age-old question that there is much debate around, as you can imagine, and there is much conflicting information available on this topic. We're talking about rubbing down that at-risk tissue between the vaginal opening and the anus in preparation for the big event. Is it helpful or just one more thing we tell each other may increase our chances of having a tear-free experience?

I'll be upfront. Physical therapy-related research shows no added benefit to perineal massage prior to labor. In the classic sense of the term, no, perineum massage will not completely prevent tearing during birth. What research[46] does recommend, however, is having internal pelvic work done to release restrictions in the coccygeus muscle as well as the levator ani muscle group, which subsequently helps release the perineum tissue.

That, of course, is if you look at the research directly addressing that question. On the other hand, looking at reproductive health in general, studies do show some possible benefits of perineal massages for labor, particularly in reducing the likelihood of tears. In a 2019 study,[47] published by the *Journal Family Reproductive Health*, researchers looked at 99 women. The perineal massages were performed during active stage labor four times, each lasting for two minutes at intervals of half an hour. The researchers found that the need for an episiotomy was significantly lower in the mothers who received massages.[47]

This issue of to massage or not to massage remains unsettled, and we can see why. It's because the issue is being viewed from many perspectives. So, while in some disciplines, it proves unhelpful, in others it just may be instrumental. In our opinion, we believe that this massage may or may not be efficient for you, it just depends on why you may need it.

Remember, all positions come with benefits and drawbacks, so whichever ones you prefer, I recommend that you discuss them with your women's health PT, healthcare provider, or birthing coach. Planning is essential, especially if you are having a rather difficult pregnancy. I'm sure you don't want a vaginal tear, after all, who does? That's why I encourage you to choose carefully and combine positioning with other practices for a safer and smoother delivery process.

WHAT WORKED FOR ME AND
MAY WORK FOR YOU TOO

When I began to plan my pregnancy, I realized that there is no shortage of information floating out there in the void of the Internet. From stuffy medical journals to "Mommy" Facebook groups, there is a place for everyone, no matter how you plan to approach pregnancy, birth, or even parenting. Finding your place, however, is the trick.

I found, for me, there was no one place where I could completely satisfy my need for education and community. I did find it very helpful when I was lost and looking for direction to engage with women who have been there and are willing to share their experiences. Their real-life birth plans, birth stories, and sage advice helped me forge my own path. In that same spirit of sisterhood, I would like to share what worked for me. My birth plan, my story, and those bits of advice I wish someone would have told me long before I experienced them myself.

My Birth Plan

A birth plan is exactly what it sounds like. It is a written declaration of your preferred birthing procedure. You can include any and all details explaining how you expect the medical professionals and hospital staff assisting you in labor and after birth to allocate your care. Your hospital or birthing center should follow your birthing plan as closely as medically possible. If there is any deviation from this plan, you should be informed at every step.

Labor, birth, and the days following are chaotic and there is a chance that you may be medicated, separated from your partner, or placed in an emergent situation. Besides directing your medical team, this plan also allows you to remember and focus when everything else may feel like it is falling apart. Being asked questions while pushing a baby out can understandably cause you to make rash decisions that you would otherwise not make in calmer times.

It is important to know that the best-laid plans can be thrown out the window. Your birth plan is a guideline and a good one to have, but if you choose to deviate, you have not failed. Your health and the health of your child is the priority on their birthday and whatever choice you make to ensure that is the right one.

Below I have included the birth plan my husband and I wrote up during my third trimester with my son. It is detailed and a culmination of my research, the advice of trusted family members and friends, and my personal wishes. It is my hope that it may help you as you draft your own, either simply as a template or as a full guide.

Pre-Labor

- As long as the baby and I are healthy, I would like to have no time restrictions on the length of my pregnancy.
- I trust that my practitioner will seek out my opinion concerning all of the issues directly affecting my birth before deviating from my plan.
- Please obtain my permission before stripping my membranes during a vaginal exam. I prefer to have only one vaginal exam on or around my due date and at no time to have my membranes broken unless there is an emergency situation.
- If induction is deemed necessary, I am open to trying the following as a primary action:
  - Breast stimulation
  - Walking
  - Acupuncture
  - Sexual intercourse

Pain Management

- Massage
- Breathing and distraction techniques
- The use of water/tub/shower
- The use of heat/ice packs
- Please only offer pain medications if I ask for them

Second Stage of Labor

- As long as the baby and I are healthy, I prefer to have no time limits on pushing.
- It's important to me to push instinctively, not wanting to be told how/when to push.
- I wish to utilize various pushing positions that feel right at the time.
- Encourage me to breathe properly for slower crowning and apply warm compresses.

Birth & Immediate Postpartum Care

- As long as my baby is healthy, I would like him placed immediately skin-to-skin on my abdomen covered with a warm blanket.
- Please wait for the umbilical cord to stop pulsating before it is clamped and allow Steven to cut the cord.
- I would prefer for the placenta to be born spontaneously without the use of pitocin, and/or controlled traction on the umbilical cord.

Newborn Care and Procedures

- If the baby has any problems, I would like my husband to be present with him at all times. Please delay all essential routine procedures on my baby until after the bonding and breastfeeding period.
- Please do not administer eye drops to my baby, I am willing to sign a formal waiver. Our baby is to be exclusively breastfed. I

would like to see a lactation consultant as soon as possible for further recommendations and guidance.

- We would like our baby circumcised.
- I prefer to have my husband stay with me for the duration of my hospital stay.
- If a cesarean becomes absolutely medically necessary, we wish to maintain as many aspects of our birth plan as possible, creating a gentle family-centered cesarean birth experience for our baby and for us.
- If a C-section is not an emergency, please give my husband and I time alone to think about it before asking for our written consent.
- I would like my husband and doula to be present at all times.
- Please discuss with me what I can expect to feel immediately following the procedure as well as my post-operative pain medication options with me before or immediately following the procedure.
- We'd like delayed cord clamping.
- I would like to have my baby shown to me immediately and to have skin-to-skin contact with him as soon as possible in the delivery room.
- I would like my husband to be the baby's constant source of attention until I am free to bond (i.e., holding, skin-to-skin contact, etc.).
- If the baby has any problems, I would like Steven to be present with him at all times, if possible.
- Please explain all procedures before and as they are performed, as the baby's condition permits if his health is in jeopardy.
- I would like all newborn routine procedures to be performed in our presence.

Thank you for your support, communication, and expert care!
Go ahead, Mama, take a breath and soften.

HOW IT WENT: LABOR, DELIVERY, AND BEYOND

The birth of my son is still fresh in my mind. Upon writing this, I am only a few weeks postpartum. The experience feels so far away now yet so close. Immortalizing it here, for you, can only be called cathartic. I hope it helps as you envision welcoming your own baby.

First things first, I needed my people and my plan. I think having a natural birth is a wonderful experience, but I also felt I did a lot of mental and physical preparation to get there. I took my own advice and really analyzed the pain management options available to me and the way I would build my support team. I wrote it all down, as you saw above in my birth plan, and made sure to understand my options.

My doula's name is Barbie. I recommend bringing a doula like Barbie onto your team, if at all possible if you want to try to have a natural childbirth. I was able to stay home longer because I would communicate with Barbie. Without her, I would have likely panicked and headed to the hospital much earlier, which could have changed my experience. At home, I was comfortable, safe, and confident and I think those feelings played a large part in achieving the birth I wanted.

I could write an entire book just about my labor and the subsequent birth. It was everything I expected and so much that I did not. It was full of emotions I cannot express fully through text and moments that will forever stay in my memory and my heart. Theodore Hayes D'Andrea entered my life and changed everything. I will try with all my might to keep this short and sweet.

I have heard hundreds of birth stories as a pelvic health specialist and my biggest takeaway was that every birth is different and beautiful and unpredictable. No two are the same. But I gained a sense of peace knowing that one of the best things I could do to prepare was to keep an open mindset, stay flexible, and roll with the punches.

One of the most variable aspects of pregnancy and birth center around that very last stretch. I heard everything from, "I gained all my weight in the last month" to "I gained no weight in the last month" to "the last 4 weeks are the worst" to "the entire third trimester is misera-ble." I was no different. If my pregnancy discomfort was a graph, it would have looked something like this: a long, steady, gradual incline, and then a sudden spike at the very end.

It was all pretty easy and comfortable, and then BOOM! I hit 37 weeks and was just over it. I felt like I was living inside this very large, swollen suit that I just wanted to take off. 37 weeks is when most doctors consider babies to be full term and they say that labor could potentially happen at any time; just knowing that 37 weeks was considered "full term" made my brain consider it some sort of a finish line, which was a mistake because it made the following days feel so long.

At 37 weeks + 4 days pregnant, I woke up and I was surprised to find blood in the toilet after urinating. My mother texted to ask how I was doing, and I responded, "I'm not sure." That's all I could articulate at the moment. My body had shown signs of going into labor, and I was desperately ready to not be pregnant. It was a Wednesday morning, and my husband, Steven, and I had plans to go to work for the day. Instead, I decided to cancel my day of patients as I knew labor was nearing and we enjoyed a lazy morning in a bed full of excitement (he watched the morning news and I read one of my Mama's natural pregnancy books). Daily bike rides were a ritual of mine during the entire pregnancy, but that morning I simply didn't have the energy for it. I felt a definite shift in my body; things were happening that signaled labor was close.

That morning, I had my bloody show and then later in the day I lost my mucus plug—two things that can often mean that labor might be near, but it could still be several days away. Just one more way that the end of pregnancy was messing with my head. I went into my clinic around 11 a.m. to chat with my team and get a few things in order that needed addressing. I found myself frantically cleaning things that I had been meaning to get to for the last few months and pacing around looking for things to organize. When I finally left the clinic, I started feeling some discomfort in my lower abdomen, but I didn't think too much of it. There are so many uncomfortable sensations at the end of pregnancy, and this crampy sort of feeling didn't seem all that special.

The feeling kept coming back again and again. I decided to time it and realized that it was lasting for about 20-30 seconds and they were happening every 15-30 minutes. Realization started to dawn, slowly. The contractions seemed pretty random, and my cynical mind just wouldn't believe this was actually the beginning of labor. I probably heard too many stories of false labors and people getting sent home from the hospital, so I tried to ignore the sensation and go on with the rest of my errands. I figured that if this was the real thing, I should try to stay calm and get as much done as possible during the early part of the day so by the time I got home I could get some rest in case labor was beginning.

Every time I tried to fall asleep, which I desperately needed, I would get nervous and begin timing again. They were fairly painless in the beginning and I was unsure if they were an indication of anything real. This went on until about 4 p.m., when I decided to open my book and go ahead and finish up the last few chapters.

I was resting on the couch and felt the urge to get up and wretch, and when I did I felt and heard a loud pop sound in my pelvis followed by feeling a gush of fluid flow from my pelvis. I went to the toilet and when I was finished I went to get up only to realize I couldn't go far—I was leaking fluid again. I sat back down on the toilet and was there for a good 30 minutes. My water had broken.

My husband called my OB's office and spoke to the midwife at the hospital to let her know what was going on. Then for the next two hours, he was a champ and ran around the house packing everything on my checklist, loading the car, running errands for me, making sure I ate something, feeding the dog, putting out the trash/recycling for trash day, and getting ready for a couple of days at the hospital. New dads sure are something special.

The weird thing about contractions is that they really are like a wave—they start very, very mild and then build to the middle to an intensity where I couldn't do anything else, even talk to someone, and then they would gradually taper off. So, it took a while to figure out when the start of each wave was happening. I didn't really time contractions until the crest of the wave when the most intense pain was there, but then I figured out to start the timer at the beginning of the wave.

Sometimes I would not realize it was happening until the pain was intense, and then all I could say was, "Help" to Steven instead of, "Can you help me get through this contraction?" He knew what I needed either way, and when I'd whimper out he'd run over from packing up the car and sway with me, breathe with me, or just put a hand on my back until the pain ended.

By the time 8 p.m. rolled around, I was in a significant amount of discomfort and didn't want to risk staying at home any longer. I was dreading the car ride to the hospital knowing how uncomfortable driving and riding in the car had been during the third trimester. Surprisingly, my back pain had gone away so I was just able to focus on the intensifying contractions. Once we arrived at the hospital we were admitted to triage fairly quickly and I learned I was already 4cm dilated.

I was relieved to hear this news and knew I wouldn't be getting sent home at this point. The nurse came in and took my vitals and right away started to set up an IV. I quickly told her that I respectfully decline having an IV, that I was staying well hydrated (I showed my 2L sized water bottle) to her. I could tell this took her by surprise, she didn't have an answer right away, until about 30 seconds later when she responded saying she'd have to run it by the doctor on staff. While I was getting checked in and answering a bunch of questions from the nurse, my doula, Barbie, walked in.

The next part is pretty boring. I just rested for about 3 hours! I was so comfy and sleepy. The lights were dimmed, I took a nap, and when I woke up I honestly couldn't remember where I was or what I was doing. The nurse would come in periodically and check on me and sometimes help me rollover, and Steven would offer me fluids. I drank a lot because I was feeling hungry and wanted some calories!

At one point my midwife came in and checked my cervix to see how dilated I was. A few hours later she checked me and I was 9.4cm, and she said she'd be back in an hour and it would be time to push! I decided to use the hot tub to help with that last bit of dilation and found it to be very relaxing, except when the contractions came, of course.

At about 9 a.m. the nurse came to prepare the room for delivery, and I found myself getting more and more vocal when the contractions came and went. I was extremely tired by this point, it had been a full day of being in pre-labor. As my body was going through transition, I started shaking uncontrollably and feeling really sick to my stomach. The shaking was due to all the hormonal changes that were taking place and my body getting ready for birth. Steven came over and let me lean my weight on him, he supported me and kept my feet grounded.

I started feeling sick to my stomach, and I asked for a barf bag just in time. I was so exhausted at one point I remember crying out to Steven saying that I wish I had chosen to have an epidural to ease the pain. I could feel my body starting to wither and mentally I felt defeated. I didn't feel like any real progress was being made. I had spent a good 30 minutes sitting on the toilet "pushing" through contractions with the midwife. I felt defeated especially there, not feeling in sync with my body, half asleep I could feel myself dozing off.

Then all of a sudden, the room got very quiet and I realized everyone had left the room with the exception of my husband. I remember asking him, "What happened? Where did everyone go?" I later learned that the medical team that was assisting me, which consisted of the midwife, two nurses, a student nurse, and my doula, had stepped out of the room to have a pow wow about my condition and how I was doing. The midwife, Linda, wanted to understand how she could better assist me and reassure me that things were progressing along just fine.

Barbie suggested that Linda take the lead so I wasn't getting different directions from five people all at once, rather just focus on one coach and have the other members assist her. This made a world of difference for me and allowed me to progress to the next phase with greater ease and confidence. So, there I was, trying every different birth position I could before the inevitable happened. Sometimes, the best-laid plans often go astray. I knew this could happen, and although I had mentally prepared for it, I still really wanted to avoid it at all costs. I found myself at a +2 station, which meant I was in a much better position to start pushing. I was supine (on my back) for the last 10 minutes or so, which in the big picture wasn't long at all. I could tell I had more power in this position and less discomfort. Had I not been at a +1 or 2 station, this position would have been more difficult and enduring for me and my baby.

I found my power and was able to connect with my breathing and pushing efforts. Despite what many people are told and what I was told to do (bear down as hard as you can like you're trying to move your bowels), I remember giving myself a gentle smile and telling myself to push while still breathing instead of holding my breath. Although it did take more time and effort, I didn't end up with hemorrhoids or a perineal tear, or worse even in my opinion, a prolapse.

I had more discomfort, more than I could possibly begin to describe, with the delivery of my placenta. The thought of the doctors is that it could have been due to the fetus that didn't make it; my placenta had adhered to my uterus and the midwife had to manually remove it, which was excruciating. I was losing a good amount of blood, to the point where my husband was noticeably getting more and more nervous by the minute. To this day, when I hear him tell friends and family about my labor journey I get choked up reliving it, all I could think is how much pain I was in, at one point I even screamed out, "Enough!"

Reflecting on it now, I am so thankful to have had such a skilled medical team working with me. I later learned the midwife was the one who actually started the midwife program at the hospital decades ago. Had it been anyone else that night, they likely would have recommended surgery to remove the placenta.

After that was over, I remember just feeling exhausted but also exhilarated. I looked at my son who was gazing directly into my eyes while laying on my chest for some skin-to-skin time and I remember thinking, *I can't believe he's here, I can't believe I did this and with no medication!* I also remember thinking, I don't know if I'd choose this route again given how awful the placenta removal was, but now that I'm a good month out, the pain is waning and I'm rethinking it! Oh, the amnesia love can cause in a mother.

I am a mother. When I hold this small body and see the curves of his father in his nose and the memories of my own eyes in his, I think about the journey that led us here. I know I am just now beginning a new one as I heal, but the gift his birth has given is neverending.

Go ahead, Mama, take a breath and soften.

From the Other Side

The following is a short antidote written by the unsung hero of our story, my husband Steven. As I researched and prepared myself for this journey, I knew that his involvement would be of the utmost importance, so it was surprising to me that I saw very little from a partner's perspective in the many books and blogs I read. It felt like there was a piece missing from the story. What did this time look like, feel like, and mean from the other side?

Well, I asked for it and you got it. Welcome to my birth story as told by the most reliable witness out there:

"Huzzy, my water just broke!" Standing there, naked, just out of the shower, I thought to myself—*wtf did she just say?* I knew some weird things were going on earlier in the morning, but off to work we went. Weird shit was par for the course throughout the pregnancy, and you learn to absorb the biological nuances of it and carry on, as they say. So we didn't think too much of it earlier that morning, or at least I didn't, and we went about our respective day.

I heard her loud, and clear; in fact it was on instant cerebral replay, but in typical male fashion I yelled back down, "What broke?!" By now I was at the top of the stairs, and she very calmly confirms what has been on instant replay upstairs, "Huzzy, my water broke." I think I might have asked something stupid, like "How do you know?" Ha. She recanted a story of a *POP!* and then something about gushing fluid. I think my next thought was, *how much time do we have?* I had a ton of things to prepare for the trip to the hospital (she had bags upon bags packed like we were headed to Europe for the Summer), and I needed to know how much time we were working with.

I probably tuned out 70% of the doula's strategy and info sessions with us—tuning into the highlights, I did recall the part about those in labor often head to the hospital too early, and I wanted to make sure we would be admitted when we got to there, so that meant laboring at home for a bit—buying me time to get us ready. Despite months of, "Steven, you need to pack your hospital bag" from my wife, I didn't have a hospital bag packed, and the car seat was still in the box! Haha, typical for sure, but the nursery was indeed squared away, so we were good there.

Now what? My wife just told me her water broke, I'm standing there in my birthday suit trying to organize the next move—"call the Doula, call the OB on call." The OB's office put us through to the midwife on duty at the hospital, and I found myself asking, when—when will I know it's time to warp speed down there?

Now we had a plan. Well, Jess is a total planner and definitely had a birthing plan, but now I felt like I had something to work with here. There was clear action, things were happening, and we had a timetable. We were looking for 2-minute intervals, and we were at a solid 20 or 30 mins. We had plenty of time. Five hours to be exact, but we didn't know that.

At this point Jess got into bed so she was as comfortable as she could be while she labored, and I raced around packing up the Jeep. We were tracking the contractions with an app the doula recommended, and Jess navigated them with what seemed to be relative ease, and I wanted to keep things as comfortable as possible. I recall thinking she was so calm, how could she be so calm—she had a tiny human in there making his way down the birth canal, and she's just chilling in bed doing her breathing exercises. She must be freaking! At one point she had me racing down to the corner store for some Depends, haha. Shortly after wrapping up with the Jeep, installing the car seat in the dark, and tossing a change of clothes in an overnight bag for myself, I checked the app and, shit—it was go time. We were averaging 2-minute contractions. I don't even remember the drive to the hospital, but I apparently got good reviews.

Boom, we were 4cm dilated, and we were being admitted! Throughout the pregnancy there are a number of little milestones that signify varying progress or a new stage. Four centimeters dilated is a massive milestone, that kid is coming! I was so consumed with caring for Jess laboring at home, and racing around getting us ready, I was in hospital mode—the reality of the event before us hadn't set in, and she was knee-deep in the middle of it. Her water broke around 5 p.m. and it was now after 11 p.m. She had been laboring for a good 6 hours, without the slightest complaint. In fact she had this calming glow about her and I was just in awe of her courage. We didn't know what was ahead of us, except Theodore was coming, that much was certain.

After some thorough due diligence from the medical team in the ER, Jess declined the initial IV. I knew that was coming, we planned for it, but I found myself internally second-guessing the plan. I was nervous for my wife, but I backed her, and after some pushback from the staff on it, they honored her wish. Our doula was onsite at this point and was able to indirectly navigate the pushback. Next stop, the ABC room—short for Alternative Birthing Center. Jess opted for a 100% holistic and natural birthing experience. She wanted a healthier experience for both herself and the boy. That happens in the ABC room.

I'm not sure what I expected of the ABC room, but as far as hospital accommodations go, this thing was impressive. We dread anything "hospital," right? There was a dedicated midwife and staff, a massive bed in the middle of the room, a private bathroom with a hot tub for laboring, a legit blanket warmer, and a ton of funny looking alternative positioning tools for laboring—but, God, was that room cold, I mean cold. She didn't notice though. Walking into the room was another one of those milestones to hit you in the face of reality, you know, in case you were still in reactive guy mode that shit was about to get real—wifey is giving birth in here. I hate to use the word "surreal," but the experience is just so surreal, every step of the way we're reminded of what we are doing—birthing a human, and it's the most frightening thing to digest. For fear of alarming Jess, I internalized a lot of those emotions. She was the star of the show, and I didn't want her experience to be any more taxing than it was about to be.

Up until this point there was what felt like a constant forward motion, a natural momentum getting us here, and then things just seemed to downshift a bit. It was this lull that brought on some defeating morale. Jess progressively labored for another 8 or 9 hours, and, boy, was the pain she was experiencing now evident. It really is what the term indicates, laboring, and more—there was a perpetual physical fight of self vs the biological process, and was it taxing. The physical and emotional toll was clearly present, and while Jess was still just so strong and positive through it, she felt defeated because she didn't feel like she was making progress. The doula had a number of great exercises to assist in the progression of labor and keep Jess's morale up while fighting for that next milestone. Ten cm dilated was what she was fighting for—ten cm dilated meant Jess could start pushing!

We were now staring at 8 or 9 a.m. and Jess was just shy of 10cm, so she hopped in the birthing tub to labor in the warm water for about an hour. In search of a more comfortable position, she moved from the tub to the toilet, yeah, the toilet, and this is when things kicked into a new gear. She was emotionally exhausted, feeling defeated, and at the height of the pain so far experienced. While I'm consoling her, I look over my shoulder, and noticed the entire staff was legit gone. Ghosted. I continued to console, coach, and reassure Jess things are good to go, but now I'm legit concerned. Later did I learn the doula took them out to the hall for a pow wow, she could see Jess was feeling defeated and needed them to get her head back into the game. With Jess still hanging on the toilet, her staff comes back in, and begins to prep the room for delivery.

While the staff preps the room, the midwife jumps in the bathroom with Jess. She gets down on her knees so she can be face-to-face with Jess. The midwife begins to coach Jess through her labor in what looked like a scene from the movie *Million Dollar Baby*. My wife was Hilary Swank and the midwife Clint Eastwood as she talked my wife through the most painful and beautiful moment of her life. Meanwhile, I stood back and stared in awe at how this mystical being (the midwife) handled the situation and made my wife so calm, even though I knew she was in excruciating pain. I did my part by holding Jess's hand and providing what comfort I could. Everything else was up to Jess at this point. When the time finally came, it was like the air in the room stood still. I held my breath as I held my wife's hand and watched Jess give one final push. With that final push, the world changed in an instant. We had a baby. A freaking tiny, adorable, red splotchy baby! I felt like giving my wife a football player's chest bump accompanied by a raucous hoot and holler. But what my wife just did was way more incredible than what any football player could ever do. My wife just had a baby, and now, I am a father.

POSTPARTUM: NOW WHAT?

irl. You did it. You gave birth. You are a mother and that tiny human who just does not seem real is here and ready to change your life completely. The hard part is over, right? All that preparation, all those expectations—all of it led to the big moment and now you are done!

Nope.

The hardest part of having a baby has just started. Postpartum has now begun, and as we said in the beginning, postpartum is forever. It is now on your body to begin repairing, realigning, and healing. Things will be strange and you will experience sensations, discomfort, and even pain that is foreign to you before now. It may even feel unfair.

I agree. What you feel, no matter what it is, is valid. Even the disconnect and the fear. You did something huge and now, you are going through giant hormonal changes and healing from a major medical event while being a caregiver. The fact that you have not dissolved into a giant puddle of tears—even if you have—is a miracle. I am proud of you. All of us are.

Let's take back control. The best thing you can do as you enter this new stage in your life is to know exactly what is happening to your body and how you can care for it as it does its thing. It is just one part of being the brave, badass, amazing woman that you are and I want to be there with you as you begin.

6 Weeks Postpartum

That just happened. Six weeks ago you and your vagina worked together to do something incredible…and painful…and messy…and, well, life-changing. You gave birth to a beautiful baby boy or girl and now, you are sitting on a doctor's exam table with an oversized piece of parchment paper sticking to the back of your legs, wondering what is next.

You are about to get the 6-week postpartum check-up talk. This is when your doctor asks you how you are feeling, how you are healing, and the dreaded, "Getting any sleep yet?" The hope is that when you slide off of the table, bits of ripped paper glued to your butt cheeks, you will be cleared to resume all of those activities you loved before giving birth. Sex, exercise, and more are officially available to you once your doctor's signature appears on the bottom of those papers. A simple process on paper.

What you might not consider is that this 6-week check-up is the debilitating anxiety you may be experiencing as your mind races through the list of strange discharges, swelling body parts, and hair loss that you told yourself you would remember to ask about as soon as you saw your doctor. Nobody mentions that you will surely forget the most important question you have been dwelling on the second the doctor opens their mouth or that you may not feel quite as ready as you are told you are.

Your 6-week postpartum check-up is about much more than getting the "all clear." This is just the beginning for you as you turn the page in the next chapter of your health. The body that worked so hard to give you the squealing bundle of joy in your arms is going to need your attention now more than ever. This begs the question—are you prepared?

What To Expect At Your 6-Week Postpartum Check-Up

Now is the time I need to just say it: if you are experiencing pain, swelling, discharge, or redness from either your C-section incision or from your stitches elsewhere, see your doctor immediately. Do not wait. Voice every and any concern you have as soon as you have it. You know your body and if you are concerned, that is reason enough to speak out. You are not ridiculous, you are not wasting your doctor's time, and at the end of the day, even if the only thing you get out of asking a question is peace of mind, that is valuable in and of itself.

Pregnancy takes a toll on your whole body, from the stuff you can see, like your skin and gut health, to the stuff you can't, like your iron levels. Every part of you is dealing with an influx of hormones and is trying to heal an injury and that feels weird and unfamiliar. When you feel like this, it helps to know exactly what to expect when you walk into your 6-week postpartum appointment.

The first thing your doctor will ask is how you are feeling; they are looking for signs that you are dealing with fatigue or postpartum depression. Mothers often think that this should be the happiest time of their life, but in reality, may be feeling anything but. Postpartum depression can creep into anyone's experience and should be treated quickly and seriously. If you have any signs that this may be affecting you, your doctor has the ability to put you in contact with someone who can help. For this reason, it is important to be as honest as possible with the doctor.

For the physical portion of the visit, the doctor will focus on your healing. Any aches and pains should be addressed now. They need to ensure you're recovering well and you're getting enough vitamins, minerals, and iron as well as healing on a visible level. If you have experienced a need for stitches, your doctor will need to perform a pelvic examination. They will look for signs of infection, such as swelling. A breast examination is another normal part of the visit. The doctor will be looking for signs of abnormalities, infection, or other issues that can accompany breastfeeding.

At this point, if you have met their expectations, your doctor may confirm that you are cleared to resume regular activity. While this may be true in the sense that you check all the boxes that indicate that you are healed to the point that it is unlikely that you will sustain a serious injury related to birth, it does not mean you, as an individual, are ready for any and everything you have on your mind.

The Myth: 6 weeks postpartum is a great time to return to running and high-impact exercise.

The Truth: It is widely accepted that many medical professionals, such as myself, recommend waiting closer to 12 weeks to resume regular activities.

This period can be shortened or lengthened depending on your personal health and anatomy as well as assistance from a pelvic floor physical therapist. As a women's health specialist and physical therapist, I can appreciate the craving to get back to your workout routine for your mental and physical health, but not at the expense of healing after birth. Being kind to yourself begins at recognizing limits and giving yourself the tools to succeed from the beginning.

That is not to say that you are stuck. There are many actions you can take to improve your strength, mobility, and stability ahead of venturing back into your regular routines. These things work in conjunction with fulfilling basic needs that often get put on the backburner when motherhood arrives. Getting adequate sleep, hydration, and good nutrition to balance out your hormones are the foundations of so much more.

The next step is figuring out why you have feelings of discomfort or pain and addressing them. Though there are many reasons, two of the most likely culprits are the pregnancy itself or even breastfeeding posture. This surprises many, but it is easy to see why breastfeeding can have an affect on the body. When you hold your baby in order to latch, it is common to round your shoulders or push them forward to compensate for the awkward positioning. This leads to tight pectorals and thoracic kyphosis. Unfortunately, this is often left unaddressed by this point of your care.

Most women walk away from their 6-week check-up with pain or discomfort and after the doctor signs off, you are alone in navigating the remainder of your recovery. If you can, ask for a referral to a pelvic health physical therapist as soon as you can. We are musculoskeletal experts and we can be your guide through some of the most difficult hurdles you will face before and after your official 6 weeks of recovery. You are a mother now, dedicated to the care and health of your new baby. Allow us to extend that same care to you and your health because that is something no one should do alone.

Is It Now OK to Work Out?

Think of pregnancy like an athletic event. At the end of the event, you may have an injury like whiplash or a really bad back injury that can take months or a full year to heal. Plan for that and start pre-habbing!

If you were to injure your knee, it is expected that you will see a physical therapist to rehab or prehab prior to surgery, if needed. You injure your ACL, and you are probably in physical therapy prior to surgery as well. The same goes for pretty much any other orthopedic surgery.

There is no stigma to preparing your body for a large medical event or facilitating preemptive healing.

Yet, if you spend 9 months lengthening your abdominal muscles, experience changes with the glutes, hips, back, and pelvic floor muscles at the minimum, there is no expectation that you will seek or receive similar care. Childbirth is a marathon on the horizon that we can anticipate. Why not begin pre-habbing for pregnancy to reduce the risk of pregnancy injury, such as diastasis recti?

Outside of physical wellbeing, bouncing back into your former figure is a common goal for new moms. The reality is, you're going to have to take things easy for a while. Your body has just performed a miracle, and the past 9 months have been an ordeal! From carrying around the additional baby weight to your skin stretching to accommodate your bundle of joy, your body is going to need time to recover and heal.

It's advised to wait for at least 6 weeks until you work out, and especially if you plan to do high-intensity exercise, such as jogging. As we discussed, this rule can, and likely will, extend to at least 12 weeks. Even if your doctor says it's OK to work out, it's important to listen to your body before hitting the gym or trying to jump back into your old workout routine.

If you ignore your body and your doctor's advice and decide to work out too early, you could cause damage to your body—something you certainly won't want to deal with as you care for a newborn. Here's what could happen if you hit the gym before you've fully recovered, to name a few:

- Urinary incontinence
- Pelvic floor prolapse
- Pelvic floor pain
- Rupture of perineal stitches if you had a perineal tear
- Improper healing of your pelvic floor and abdominal tissues

The point is to take your time. You have forever to heal. This stage of your life requires a steady and loving hand as you journey through it and that applies to the physical aspect of recovery as well as the emotional. Okay now, say it with me:

Go ahead, Mama, take a breath and soften.

IS YOUR C-SECTION CAUSING YOU PAIN?

I f you birthed your baby or babies through a cesarean, you are a strong mama. Now repeat that to yourself.

"I am a strong mama because I birthed through cesarean."

One of the most nerve-wracking things about labor is not knowing what to expect and feeling like you have no control over your own body. It's a scary prospect because many women feel like they will wake up in labor and suddenly know everything there is to know about giving birth. However, almost no one knows exactly how their labor will progress until it starts happening for them. This means that there are lots of surprises when it comes to childbirth: some good and some bad. One big surprise that many moms don't anticipate ahead of time is having a cesarean section (or C-section).

A C-section involves making an incision through the abdominal wall and uterus during delivery. To diagnose the necessity of this delivery, your doctor will monitor the fetal heart rate throughout labor. If it falls into a concerning pattern or doesn't recover after regulated contractions, you may need to have a C-section. In addition, sometimes, women who go into labor with scar tissue from previous cesareans can end up needing an emergency C-section. This is why doctors typically won't automatically schedule your baby's delivery if you've had one in the past without complications.

Let's talk about some of the truths that you may not have heard from other healthcare practitioners when it comes to this amazing, difficult thing that you did. Cesarean births, just like vaginal births, can leave us with unresolved emotions and unexpected physical setbacks. I have seen many women in my treatment room who have silently suffered for years with postpartum abdominal pain, pelvic pain, painful intercourse, low back pain, urinary leaking and urinary urgency to name a few. The thing is, there is a misconception that pelvic floor physical therapy is *only* for moms who birthed vaginally.

Often, women who have given birth by cesarean are not asked about their postpartum symptoms because there is a slightly less chance that they will end up with the symptoms listed above. I don't want your symptoms to go unnoticed. Possible cesarean birth postpartum symptoms can include: abdominal pain, hip and low back pain, urinary incontinence, urinary frequency and urgency, scar pain and numbness, pelvic and clitoral pain, and weak core muscles.

A cesarean birth is a natural birth, no less and no more than vaginal birth. This is not the easy way out, it is major surgery. There are many reasons why you may need a C-section. The below is not an exhaustive list, but includes some of the most common reasons a pregnant woman may require a C-section:

- A baby that is breech, meaning feet or butt first instead of head first.

- The umbilical cord is wrapped around the baby's neck.
- The placenta blocks the opening of the cervix (placenta previa).
- Failure to progress in labor after active efforts have been made to help the cervix dilate.
- Excessive bleeding during pregnancy, making an operation essential for the mother or baby's sake.
- The baby is showing signs of an abnormal fetal heart rate or distress.
- Maternal complications, such as high blood pressure, entering labor with a small pelvis, and previous C-sections can cause a doctor to diagnose a condition requiring immediate delivery.

Your practitioner can tell you if a planned cesarean is the best course of action for your specific situation. In addition, your doctor or midwife's rates for cesarean sections can give you a better idea of how risky your pregnancy may be. If they have an accurate NTSV (nulliparous term singleton vertex) rate, this is more likely to indicate the risks involved in having one yourself. But even if not, it will still help provide valuable insight into potential outcomes and their likelihoods so that all options may be considered before making any decisions about delivery type.

If your doctor determines that a cesarean section is necessary, you can still control some risks by taking certain precautions. For example, one way to reduce the risks is by giving birth in a hospital or surgical center, so you have access to better equipment and immediate care in case something goes wrong. Also, avoid being overweight or obese for your height if at all possible. Diabetes, high blood pressure, excessive weight gain, gestational hypertension/preeclampsia, fetal growth retardation, postpartum hemorrhage after a previous birth, delayed pushing during labor, and lacerations are also complications to be aware of as you assess your chances of having a cesarean section.

In addition to the physical risks of cesarean delivery, as mentioned above, some pretty hefty psychological expectations come along for the ride. For example, mommies with scarred uteri can develop anxiety or panic attacks around their upcoming birthdays if they have had previous C-sections. Many equate those numbers with death or dying in general. So please keep these things in mind as you go through your pregnancy planning process.

Of course, there is one other person at the top of your mind as you plan. The risk to the baby is higher when a cesarean section must be performed, but other factors can increase this as well. These risks include congenital disabilities, an increase in breathing problems at birth, increased risk of bleeding in the brain (intracranial hemorrhage), and developmental delays or learning disabilities later on.

These risks are just that—risks. Having a C-section does not guarantee your baby will be any less healthy than a baby born via vaginal birth. You and your child will, in all likelihood, be happy and healthy at the end of the day. Education should bring with it the reassurance that you are prepared, not fear. The method by which your baby enters the world is only the first of many stages they will go through to become the amazing, happy person you will raise. Remember that.

Because a C-section is major abdominal surgery, it carries its own set of risks and complications besides what we've already discussed. In addition, those who have cesareans also need to be aware that there is a higher risk for infection in the uterus or abdomen following any abdominal surgery, injury to other organs such as the bowel, bladder, ureters (tubes between bladder and kidneys), major blood vessels in the area, pelvic bone, and nerves, hernias (a bulge or lump which may cause pain) in the wound after surgery, scarring of tissue due to inflammation/infections, and problems with postoperative discomfort when moving around after surgery, including increased pain and gas pains.

After the surgery, you and your baby are further at risk for breathing problems for the baby at birth due to decreased lung maturity (inability to breathe on their own) or difficulty with the delivery itself, bleeding in the brain for both you and your child when too much blood is lost during surgery when it cannot be quickly replaced, intestinal problems are more common when there are lacerations/cuts during surgery, uterine infection is more likely in mommies who have had previous surgeries since scar tissue provides an easier entry point for harmful bacteria. A higher rate of re-hospitalization following your discharge from the hospital is also recognized as a leading risk.

Moms who have had a cesarean section may also develop pelvic pain as well as chronic pelvic pain that radiates into the lower back during their lifetime due to problems with scar tissue formation in the pelvis. Scarring increases with each subsequent cesarean delivery, so moms who have had repeated surgeries are at even more risk for these chronic problems later on.

After Your C-section

It may not feel like it directly after you undergo the surgery, but you will feel better very soon. You also are not destined to have cesarean sections with all of your subsequent pregnancies. In fact, you have quite a few options.

Deciding if this is the right choice for your next pregnancies comes with an assessment of both the risks and benefits between you and your doctor. A repeat C-section can be a relatively safe procedure with very minimal risk of a mommy dying. There are no long-term effects on fertility, menstruation patterns, or the ability to become pregnant again and the recovery time is shorter as the incision from this type of surgery heals quickly. You can labor and recover at home instead of being in an unfamiliar environment surrounded by strangers. No IV lines are required, which can make you uncomfortable during labor in many cases and there are some risk-reducing benefits for the baby as well.

On the other hand, this means that there is a need for another major abdominal surgery along with all of the risks and complications that came with your first C-section. In some instances, it also means you now have the inability to have future vaginal deliveries. You should be aware of the increased risk of infection and decrease in blood flow through the uterine wall, which may lead to fetal distress during labor. If you do not have a successful epidural placement during vaginal birth, you may be at risk for the above complications. Less bladder control after surgery can result in incontinence later on and decreased bowel function with fewer sensations of needing a bowel movement is usually associated with C-sections. These are both long-term ramifications.

Baby-wise, there is a higher chance that your child will experience respiratory distress during birth because there will be an increased amount of fluid at the time of delivery compared to vaginal births, where this complication does not often occur. There is an increased risk of the development of postpartum depression, especially if you have had previous miscarriages or infertility issues after getting home and your pelvic muscles must repair themselves after a long recovery time before returning to the strength/structure support system.

The decision to have a third C-section should depend on the family's needs and preferences. If multiple children are planned, medical authorities recommend two as max before resorting to fertility treatments such as in vitro fertilization (IVF) or egg donation.

Vaginal births after cesarean sections are often called VBAC. Statistically, it is a safer option than having an elective repeat C-section due to the lower risk of uterine rupture or problems with blood flow, but there are great benefits as well.[48] The recovery time for a VBAC is often shorter than having another C-section because the recovery from vaginal delivery is less complicated by nature. After surgery, you maintain more control over your bladder, making it easier for you to empty your bladder as well.

The Recovery Process

Many first-time moms who give birth via a C-section say they feel very vulnerable since they were not able to experience the birth they may have imagined. Emotionally and physically, it is a difficult path.

Your recovery process is different from that of vaginal births and should be treated as such. You are experiencing major surgery. For many of us, this may even be our first time under the knife. Now, in addition to recovering from birth, you are trying to heal in other ways. First, your abdominal muscles must repair themselves before returning to their supportive strength and structural support system since there was a cut in the lower left side of your body. Stitches are required to repair it and those, too, must be addressed.

Second, the birth canal was not used for delivery, so the uterus contracts back down to its original size and returns fully within one month after surgery. Women who have had C-sections often complain about having more back pain and discomfort due to the location where the incision site is made (lower part of abdomen instead of uterus).

Related to this, women also experience frequent urination, constipation, and gas pains after this procedure. Now that the bladder is empty, these symptoms that were common during their pregnancy become extremely obvious now that they are caused by surgery rather than the pressure of their baby. The incision location also presents discomfort if placed on the lower abdomen. Some women complain about standing up straight or sitting up straight because there is some pain associated with these movements.

The risk of uterine infection is arguably the most dangerous aspect of recovery. In the unfortunate case that you do suffer from an infection, you might require IV antibiotics after surgery. In addition, fluid may build up around or on top of your incision site if it heals poorly (called a seroma), but this usually goes away within six months without treatment. If you notice excessive swelling, redness, warmth extended beyond one inch above the incision line, and fluid drainage from the incision site beyond six weeks postpartum, you must contact your doctor immediately.

Some parts of your recovery do remain the same, of course. Namely, nourishing your body, which has gone through so much. Food may not be the first thing on your mind after getting home due to a lack of stomach distention (from pregnancy), which causes nausea. You have to get something down though! Breastfeeding moms must eat extra protein in order for milk production to increase along with calcium intake through foods or supplements so you can produce enough milk for your baby. Eating healthy foods will be a vehicle for a healthy recovery as well as a great start for your breastfeeding journey.

Long after you begin to feel recovered, your scar will be obvious. The appearance of your scar should be flat after a year or more, but takes a lifetime for the skin to become smooth again. So, even though the scar may appear healed, your skin may not feel "normal" until you have lost all of your weight gained during pregnancy. Even then, it may be tough to recognize your body as your own.

Physically, this process causes an increase in abdominal tension, which pulls on the wound site, making it very uncomfortable for you. It can take 6-9 months postpartum before this becomes less of an issue. Depending on your comfort level, it is just fine to wait 6 months before you start exercising again. In fact, it may be prudent to wait this long as intense exercise causes sweating, which increases the risk of infection. This is why walking is so important after this particular surgery. Many women find walking more comfortable than strenuous exercise because it reduces the risk of infection. It also helps relax your muscles, speeds up the healing process, and is easy on your wound site since there is less pressure from jostling. Walking doesn't require any special equipment other than a good pair of walking shoes to help prevent injury, so this makes it an excellent first step towards getting back into shape.

Once you are more comfortable discovering your personal exercise limits, go slowly. You should definitely wait at least six weeks before you can even think about lifting anything heavier than 20 pounds (most household items) since this increases abdominal tension, which can cause complications during wound healing. Traditional crunches are not recommended either because they increase intraabdominal pressure that pulls on the wound site, so focus on abdominal compression exercises, like the pelvic tilt. This reduces intra abdominal pressure and thus takes stress off the wound site. Avoid any activities that cause you to perspire heavily, such as aerobics and jogging. These activities increase infection risk, which could be deadly, especially during the first month when your wound is most vulnerable to infection.

After listing all of these risks and complications in one place, it is easy to see why many women experience pain months after having a cesarean section, without realizing that it is directly related to that surgery and that they need to seek treatment. Every mom who has a cesarean birth deserves postpartum physical therapy. Chances are, PT wasn't offered to you postpartum. It is not commonly known that women's health physical therapists are able to help you rehab and return to exercise safely following a cesarean birth. If you don't feel like "yourself" after a cesarean, you are not alone!

Note: some medical offices offer "physical therapy," but you are actually just strapped to a biofeedback machine and a med tech (without a graduate degree) tells you to Kegel and relax. THIS IS NOT pelvic floor physical therapy and it 100% will not help you get better. Instead, look to someone that treats your body as a whole after taking the time and effort to truly understand it.

Story form a Sister: Sofia

Sophia is a 45-year-old busy mother of three children under the age of 10. She had been dealing with bladder leakage as well as rectal prolapse since she gave birth to her first child. Sophia loves to work out and weight training. Running was an especially favorite hobby in her past. All in all, Sophia was a fit woman who did everything she could to stay that way before and after her pregnancies.

That is not to say that she was without physical issues. Before going on a run, Sophia was used to peeing "just in case" before leaving the house. She was experiencing symptoms of increased pressure and heaviness in her pelvic floor, but pushed the concern to the back of her head. She, like many of my pelvic health patients, thought that this was just what happens after having children. This resulted in her attempting to rectify her issues on her own.

Sophia tried some Kegel exercises for a few weeks and was surprised they did not help her symptoms one bit. One day, it came to a head when she went for a run and came back soaked from having lost control of her bladder. This is when she began to seek help. Sophia spoke with various physicians and got several different opinions on what her next step should be. The only thing these suggestions had in common was that they would result in surgery, whether it was to input mesh for the prolapse or a pessary for her bladder.

Sophia decided to take her health into her own hands and do her own research. She decided to see if a pelvic health specialist could help her heal naturally and get her back to her favorite exercises, like running for at least 10 miles without leaking. She also wanted to just be able to go to a store without having to map out her route based on where the bathrooms were. She came to Arancia PT full of hope and encouragement and within 11 sessions, she had met her goal. She is now back to running 10+ miles a day with no leaking and has found at least 20 minutes a day to devote just to herself for self-care and treatment. She even comes in once a month for tune ups to keep up her amazing progress. The best part, Sophia never had to go under the knife to do it.

PELVIC ORGAN PROLAPSE

I believe every newly postpartum mama should be equipped with the right questions at your 6-week postpartum follow-up appointment. One of these questions is, "Am I at risk of a pelvic organ prolapse?"

Most OBGYNs are well aware of how to assess for pelvic organ prolapse or POP. However, that does not mean that they actually perform POP assessments. Though there may be several reasons that the assessment is neglected, I truly believe that the real reason is that physicians can be very limited on time when it comes to individual patient care. In an insurance-driven system, this means that time is money.

A basic questionnaire will weed out a large portion of patients who do not need additional care so many choose to save time and money by doing the minimum. For those of us that this is sufficient for, there is no problem and they stay on track with their time. For those of us whom this is not sufficient, we are left to navigate the issues alone. If they do happen to assess a new mother and find that she does have some degree of prolapse, options for treatment are limited. 90% of cases never end up under the care of a physical therapist[49], much less a physical therapist who specializes in pelvic health.

Mama's, this is not okay! If we have a POP diagnosis, it is extremely helpful to see a pelvic floor physical therapist to learn how to manage symptoms, if there are any. POP is scary and you should not deal with it alone. From the way that you take in breaths to proper exercise of the tissue and muscles, everything should be guided by an expert. We want to see you get better for the long term.

If you experience POP, don't freak out! The majority of women end up with POP at some point in their lives. Being aware and informed is the first step in managing your diagnosis. As you complete this chapter, you will be exactly that. Welcome to everything you need to know about POP from a medical professional who sees and treats at least 10 women diagnosed with POP a week!

What is POP?

POP is defined as the hernia of organs in the pelvic region to the vaginal opening. Imagine your pelvis is divided into the three main organs: the bladder, the uterus, and the rectum. These organs are supported and kept in place by an intricate support network of muscles that act like a hammock, cradling them and keeping them in the correct position. This hammock-style support network comprises several muscles, fibers, and ligaments that work in conjunction to keep these organs safe. If, for any reason, this support network is damaged or is weakened, these organs can descend from their intended position and drop into the vagina. This becomes your POP.

POP can either be symptomatic or asymptomatic. If the pelvic floor muscles are weakened or damaged but the organs are not past the vaginal opening, then women who suffer from POP might not experience any symptoms at all and will be described as asymptomatic. But if the pelvic floor muscles are significantly damaged and the organs start to protrude from the vaginal opening, then there can be some complications. This will be classified as symptomatic pelvic organ prolapse.

According to data, more than 200,000 pelvic organ prolapse surgeries take place in the US annually.[50] POP is not a fatal condition. It does, however, affect the quality of life for women in a significant way and results in many major lifestyle changes. Anything that affects your ability to function normally is important and should be treated as such.

It can be scary to learn that you might have POP, but it is crucial that you seek medical advice as soon as you can. Hiding from your condition is not the solution. Many women tend to keep the problem a secret and end up suffering in secret as well. When it becomes too much, the only solution may be drastic. Speak up and seek medical advice so that you can do your best to avoid unnecessary surgery.

What Are the Stages of POP?

There are four stages of pelvic organ prolapse. Each stage comes with its own concerns and possible treatment. Even if you find that your POP is easily managed, knowing exactly what you are dealing with allows you to make safe and informed decisions about your care.

Stage 1—This is considered a mild or mostly harmless stage of a POP. In this stage, the pelvic floor is just starting to lose its strength but is strong enough to provide ample support to the organs. There are usually no symptoms during this stage, and you are unlikely to experience any major discomfort.

Stage 2—This stage is when the POP starts to reach a more advanced state. The pelvic floor keeps losing strength and the pelvic floor organs start to descend. During this stage, they are still inside the vagina. Some symptoms can start to show during this stage, but many women do not experience any symptoms at all.

Stage 3—This is the stage where the POP starts to become severe. The pelvic organs fall into the vagina or past its opening. Most women experience symptoms during this stage.

Stage 4—This is the last and most severe stage of POP. The pelvic organs complete their descent and protrude through the vaginal opening. This is what most people think of when they think of POP. You cannot ignore this stage without suffering discomfort or pain.

What Causes POP?

As we have previously mentioned, pelvic organ prolapse occurs when the supporting tissues, such as ligaments, are damaged or weakened allowing for the uterus to descend into the vagina. Damage to supportive tissue can occur in multiple ways, but the most common is pregnancy.

Pregnancy, by its nature, requires all sorts of stretching and distress in the pelvic area and most women incur POP to some degree postpartum. The chances of the supporting tissue in the pelvic floor being weakened or damaged increase in the case of triplets or twins. Multiple pregnancies are also a common cause of this problem. Sometimes, a natural vaginal childbirth that is rushed can also cause the pelvic floor to take damage. If the baby is large or the mother has to go through a rough pushing phase chances of POP increase as well.

Outside of pregnancy, there are multiple causes as well. Obesity can cause intra-abdominal pressure to be exerted on the pelvic floor, which weakens it and over time the pelvic floor is damaged. Constipation is an unlikely culprit as well. Women who have trouble passing bowel movements on the toilet and strain a lot can develop pelvic organ prolapse. The straining puts pressure on the pelvic floor weakening the muscles.

After a woman goes through menopause her estrogen levels start to drop, which is also a known factor that can cause POP. Even women who suffer from asthma or chronic bronchitis who are prone to severe coughing may find themselves experiencing POP. When you cough repeatedly with high intensity, it exerts a tremendous amount of intra-pressure on your pelvic floor. This can result in damaging the connective tissue and cause POP. Other conditions, like pelvic tumors and fibroids, can also be the cause of POP.

How Do I Know if I Am Experiencing POP?

Pelvic organ prolapse is a tricky health concern with tricky symptoms. Many women report no symptoms at all until the problem becomes severe. Without symptoms, POP becomes difficult to diagnose. If you do experience symptoms, they can be very useful in detecting your POP at an early and easily-managed stage. Here are some of the common symptoms that are reported by women suffering from pelvic organ prolapse:

- A feeling of fullness or pressure in their pelvic region.
- A mild or severe backache that seems to be affecting the lower back area.
- Many women have reported that they experience pain when having sexual intercourse.
- An uneasy feeling as if something is coming out of the vagina. It can feel similar to sitting on a ball.
- There can also be a feeling of heaviness in your genitals or the lower area of the stomach.
- A visible lump or bulge in the vagina.

- Problems while peeing. It can feel like your bladder is not fully empty. You might find yourself going to use the restroom more often. Urine can start to leak when you sneeze or cough.

It is important to remember here that sometimes women do not experience any symptoms at all. This is why it is crucial to work towards maintaining the health of your pelvic muscles.

How Do I Treat My POP?

There are several forms of treatment for POP. Both surgical and non-invasive options can help treat the condition. It is advised to seek professional medical advice from your doctor regarding which mode of treatment will be the most effective for you.

1. Physical Therapy – As we mentioned earlier, oftentimes the cause of POP is the weakening of the pelvic floor muscles. Although they are weak, that doesn't mean that strengthening is our first priority. Instead, we must treat tissue that has become hypertonic or too tight. We do this through release work, which will address pain, inflammation, and alignment so that when it does come time for targeted strengthening, you are strengthening in an optimal alignment, rather than reinforcing a dysfunctional one.

2. Pessaries for POP – Pessaries are medical devices made of silicone that can be used to provide support to the pelvic organs if the pelvic floor muscles are damaged or weakened. Pessaries are inserted into the vagina and secured with a Valsalva. They are very potent at dealing with the symptoms of POP. Medical professionals can help create a custom pessary according to the

shape and size of your body. Your pessary needs to be comfortable above all else since you will be using it on a daily basis. You will also need to remove it for maintenance and cleaning. Your doctor may also prescribe vaginal estrogen to provide lubrication and comfort. It will also help lower the chances of any UTI infections.

3. Surgery – This should be the ultimate last resort! If you have tried physical therapy already with a women's health specialist and have not had success and your prolapse is more severe, then this could be something to consider. There are five surgical options that can help you treat POP. Your doctor will be able to guide you with which option will work best in your case. Here are the surgical options that can help treat POP:

   o Cystocele Repair – If your urethra or bladder has prolapsed, then this surgery will repair them.
   o Rectocele Repair – If your small bowel or rectum have prolapsed, then this surgery will repair them.
   o Hysterectomy – This surgery involves the removal of your uterus.
   o Vaginal Obliteration – This surgery will close your vagina.
   o Vaginal Vault Suspension – This surgery will repair your vaginal wall.

Rebeccas's Story

Believe it or not, sometimes symptoms of issues that may become unbearable after birth often begin before you even become pregnant. Rebecca is a patient of mine who began pelvic health therapy at my clinic after trying various different diets, supplements, and other holistic treatment approaches to treat GI issues. The problems at the time were fairly manageable and stemmed from holding bowel movements for extended periods of time, forcing her to become irregular and giving her abdominal pain and distention. Besides this, Rebecca is a generally healthy and fit 24-year-old with a job that keeps her on her feet.

She is also a mom of a beautiful two-year-old little girl, which leads to how I met her. Rebecca's first few remarks to me were that she is so frustrated with her postpartum experience that she doesn't see herself having any more children. She reported feeling vulnerable and no longer confident during intercourse as she no longer feels the same sensation with penetration that she used to. She was also highly vulnerable and embarrassed about the occasional anal leakage that happens randomly throughout the day so she is no longer comfortable trying a variety of different positions with her partner.

Embarrassed to talk about her symptoms with friends and family, she's resorted to online social media groups for some room to vent to others who could hopefully understand what she's dealing with.

Let us backtrack, just a tad. When she was at the hospital in the labor and delivery room with her daughter, things were progressing quite slowly, which can be common with first-time moms. However, things took a quick turn when Rebecca overheard the two nurses in her room whispering that the baby's heart rate was dropping. Of course, this created increased tension and anxiety for Rebecca. On her next contraction, the nurses told her to push. She did so, so hard that the vessels in her face were becoming visible. Rebecca reported many times not being able to feel if anything was happening. This is common when having an epidural, as you can lose the connection between you and your body when the medication numbs your body. Her baby was born healthy and with no concern after that last, forceful push, however, Rebecca would not be the same from that point on. She had extreme pain while sitting and with bowel movements. Most upsetting, she reported leakage of brown-tinged mucus, and occasionally blood, from her anus. She was often constipated and experienced pain when she was able to move her bowels. Upon examination, she had a bulge or the appearance of a small, skin-colored mass that extended outside her anus.

In addition, she didn't feel completely empty after a bowel movement. Rebecca had a habit of holding her breath and using all her might when asked to contract her pelvic floor muscle group. As a provider, I've never seen someone exert so much effort to try and engage their pelvic floor muscles. She simply could not tell or feel the connection to what she was doing. Had she come in pre-pregnancy, or even during pregnancy, the plan would start right away. We would have begun teaching her effective breathing methods, toileting methods, body awareness, postural and sleep corrections and we would have begun to address her pelvic malalignment as well as the tension in her sacrum and rectum.

Oftentimes, medical providers in the traditional western medicine realm are rushed due to the limitations of time and the number of patients they are expected to care for. I believe wholeheartedly that this type of scenario could have been avoided altogether if more time was taken to explain the importance of breathing to Rebecca. At her visits, there was more time for Rebecca to discuss her toileting habits and GI issues from the past and recommendations were given for pelvic health physical therapy as well as doula services.

Doulas can be wonderful assets to moms and dads during labor and the time leading up to labor. They act on behalf of the parents to provide additional support, encouragement, a voice for you to speak up to the doctors should you need anything, including any interventions, etc. Most importantly, they keep you and your partner calm!

After Rebecca's first visit with us, she already reported feeling so much better the next day feeling hopeful for the first time since this all began! She reported less sacral/rectal pain and with her first bowel movement since treatment she reported feeling completely empty! For all reading this, this could be you, and know there is hope. There is a solution that does not have to involve medication, injections and/or surgery. Knowledge is power. Applied knowledge is power!

Let us all share this knowledge with our fellow sisters, mothers, daughters, and friends so no one has to go through unnecessary pain, embarrassment, fear, shame, or doubt. Rebecca went from feeling insecure with her partner during intercourse after having her baby, to finally feeling like there is an end in sight soon to her current bowel issues. Every patient is very different and heals differently. Allow your body time to heal, seek out a pelvic health specialist near you, and do your research. You owe it to yourself to feel your best and enjoy postpartum life!

UNDERSTANDING TAILBONE PAIN DURING PREGNANCY AND POSTPARTUM

During pregnancy, you will likely be uncomfortable. You may even experience persistent pain. One such is coccyx pain. In simpler words, it is the pain you feel in your tailbone. It is not uncommon, but when you are on your butt recovering, it can be one of the most annoying!

I had significant tailbone pain, which lasted a good seven weeks after giving birth to my son, Teddy. The pain I experienced was significant, and at times made sitting unbearable. I was only able to get comfortable laying on my side. Let me tell you, being restricted in movement after birth is terrible, but it can be helped. So, if your tailbone has become a real pain in the butt, keep reading!

What is the Coccyx or Tailbone?

The coccyx is popularly known as the tailbone; it is a very tiny bone at the bottom of your sacrum. Your sacrum is the triangular bone at the end of your lumbar vertebrae (your backbone). The coccyx is basically the vestigial tail of humans, which disappears during the 8th week of pregnancy. It joins the pelvis at the sacrum bottom and this connection is called sacrococcygeal symphysis, which is further supported by five ligaments. It is because of these connections that most of your movements are pain-free.

The coccyx is additionally supported by a lot of small muscles, which is very significant for the body to function optimally. Thus, this tiny bone has a huge role in the normal functioning of the pelvic region and that is explained below. Also, the connection between the coccyx and the pelvic floor allows it to acquire different positions in men and women. For instance, it points anteriorly in men but downward in women. Well, this is very beneficial as it provides some extra space for the baby in the body so that the mother can hold it right.

The coccyx is one of the most significant parts of your lower body, especially during pregnancy. For instance, the tailbone and the ischium, which is the bony part of the butt, provide a tripod support system that is very important while you are sitting. It distributes your weight evenly and ensures the balance and stability of the region. Furthermore, the coccyx connecting to the muscles in the pelvic floor plays a great role in its stability and strength.

This helps you walk, run, and move around easily. Also, the tailbone is important because it supports the anus and vagina for easy excretion. Because your tailbone aids with connecting your pelvic floor muscles and also with balance, during pregnancy it supports the muscles that hold your uterus (womb) in place too. This is essential since your baby is within your uterus until birth.

Tailbone Pain During and After Pregnancy

Tailbone pain during pregnancy and postpartum is very common for multiple reasons. As mentioned above, women go through a lot of changes in their bodies during childbirth. One of those changes is the low back curve. It is commonly experienced by pregnant women when they stand or tuck their butt or clench their glutes, their low back curve increases.[51] The body's center of gravity also changes and women lose their core strength as well. The abdominal muscles stretch to a great extent to make more room for the baby, which is likely to cause tailbone pain. The next reason could be the position of the baby. If your baby is posterior (positioned headway down), its head is likely to push against your sacrum and tailbone. It adds to the pressure on the two, leading to discomfort and pain.

Your pelvic floor is greatly affected during the birth of your baby. This is the reason for postpartum tailbone pain (pain after delivery). There is a muscle called levator ani muscle and it is responsible for coccyx attachment and is closely related to the prolapse of the pelvic organ. The use of forceps during vaginal delivery can lead to tearing away of this muscle among up to 50% of women.[52] A part of the muscle is likely to pull off from the pubic bone and may cause tailbone pain. Also, during vaginal delivery, the muscles and ligaments stretch and destabilize your lower back, sacrum, and coccyx. This stretching and overstretching is another reason for tailbone pain after pregnancy. Additionally, the use of epidural during the delivery process is also linked with lower back pain. Finally, the mother acquires some stressed positions while delivering the baby. This is one of the factors for tailbone pain as it undergoes major pressure and stress to facilitate the passage of your baby.

What Can Be Done to Help Coccyx Pain During Pregnancy & Postpartum?

The first thing you need to do is consult a pelvic health physical therapist and get some therapy. Pelvic floor training can help you ensure stability, mobility, and enhanced coordination. It can help your coccyx to position right so that you can hold your baby easily. I would urge you to find a therapist who is trained at treating the pelvic floor internally as well as externally. Releasing the pelvic tissues internally can be highly effective for tailbone pain.

More specifically, myofascial release, dry needling, acupuncture, and visceral mobilization are some other therapies you can acquire to relieve your tailbone pain. Besides this, fixing your lifestyle can also help with the situation. Make sure to keep a neutral spine while sitting, standing, resting, etc. Eat healthily and work out. Posture is key and being aware of how you hold your body will decrease a great deal of your discomfort.

Diaphragmatic breathing can also help you with the situation. It helps in creating appropriate pressure in the abdomen and helps with bowel health by acting as a continuous massage, helps to alleviate the low back pain, and naturally stretches and strengthens the pelvic floor.

EVERYTHING YOU
NEED TO KNOW ABOUT
POSTPARTUM DEPRESSION

The birth of a baby brings with it loads of excitement, joy, love, and blessings. But it also brings with it fear, anxiety, and sometimes even depression. We call this postpartum depression.

Postpartum literally means "after childbirth." Many women experience baby blues after delivering their baby, but these symptoms usually resolve on their own within the first week. However, if the feeling persists for more than two weeks, it is called postpartum depression. It is a serious mental illness, and you should take care of yourself to prevent it from developing into psychosis.[53]

Postpartum depression is not a flaw or weakness of any sort—it is simply a complication associated with childbirth. PPD includes physical, behavioral, and emotional changes that women might experience after giving birth. It is a major form of depression and usually starts around a month after delivery. These changes are probably due to the social, chemical, hormonal, and psychological changes the parents experience when having a baby.[54]

Stats reveal that almost one in every nine women[53] and one in every ten men[55] experience postpartum depression after having a baby. And of these new moms, almost 1 in 1,000 develop postpartum psychosis.[54]

What Are Baby Blues?

Women feel a strong sense of sadness once their baby is out of their womb. This emptiness is accompanied by mood swings, crying spells, anxiety, irritability, a loss of appetite, reduced concentration, and sleep problems. Nevertheless, it usually only lasts about 3 to 5 days after the delivery and does not pose significant health risks.[53,56] However, if these symptoms last longer than a week or two, you should probably get screened for PPD.

Symptoms of Postpartum Depression

The symptoms of postpartum depression are far more intense and longer-lasting than baby blues, and thus, they tend to interfere with your life, causing further distress.

These signs include:

- Excessive crying
- Mood swings
- Loss of appetite or eating excessively
- Overwhelming fatigue
- Inability to bond with your baby
- Insomnia or over-sleeping

- Sense of hopelessness
- Irritability and anger
- Reduced interest in things you used to love
- Restlessness
- Withdrawing from family and friends
- Severe anxiety and panic attacks
- Inability to concentrate, think clearly, or make decisions
- Feeling like you're not a good mother
- Feeling worthless, ashamed, guilty, or inadequate
- Having thoughts about harming your baby
- Recurring thoughts of death and suicide

These symptoms may vary in different women, both in severity and duration.[56] In rare cases, the symptoms might worsen over time and eventually develop into a more permanent form of depression, which we call postpartum psychosis. The signs and symptoms of this condition include:

- Obsessive thoughts about your baby
- Excessive energy and agitation
- Confusion and disorientation
- Delusions and hallucinations
- Paranoia
- Sleep disturbances
- Attempting to harm yourself or your baby

This state can be life-threatening, and patients must seek immediate treatment to avoid further complications.[56]

New fathers also go through PPD, wherein they might experience some of the following symptoms:

- Overwhelming fatigue
- Anxiety

- A drastic change in appetite
- Unusual changes in sleeping pattern

These depressive symptoms are pretty much the same as those experienced by new moms. Nonetheless, fathers with a previous history of depression or greater stress levels will likely experience more severe anxiety and PPD.

How to Prevent PPD?

Some people have a higher risk of PPD than others, especially if they have a history of depression. Hence, if you're pregnant or planning a pregnancy, make sure you tell your doctor in advance so that they can advise you appropriately. During your pregnancy, you will need to be monitored for symptoms of depression. Plus, you might need counseling, support groups, or therapy to manage some of these symptoms. In fact, your doctor might even prescribe antidepressants while you are pregnant. And once your baby is out, you'll need to get checked for postpartum symptoms and maybe even begin treatment immediately because the earlier the condition is diagnosed, the better you can manage it.[54]

When to Consult a Doctor?

If you think you are suffering from postpartum depression, you should actively seek out treatment as soon as possible because if left untreated, it will only become worse. Besides adversely affecting the mental health of new moms and dads, the illness can jeopardize their relationship with their baby and also cause other family problems. The constant emotional stress can take a serious toll on the parents' health, even if only one of the two partners is affected because their dismal state is bound to influence their other half as well. And through it all, the child is likely to be neglected and thus, develop behavioral, emotional, and developmental problems of their own. They might also have trouble eating or sleeping, and much like their affected parents, they will often cry without reason.[56]

Apart from depression, PPD can also make you feel ashamed, embarrassed, or guilty—as if you are to blame for what is happening. You don't know what's wrong with you. You want to feel happy, but you don't, and you don't want other people to find out what you're thinking and feeling. You want to put on a brave face and just let it pass. But sadly, it doesn't work that way. PPD is very dangerous, and sooner or later, you will need to consult a professional.

You know it's time to call the doctor, when:

- Symptoms last more than two weeks
- The condition is hindering your daily routine
- Symptoms start getting worse
- You cannot take care of yourself or your baby
- You have thoughts about hurting your baby

Your doctor, nurse, or midwife will ask questions and screen for depression before declaring you a PPD patient.[53]

How is Postpartum Depression Diagnosed?

When you visit your doctor, they will probably discuss your thoughts and feelings to determine your current state of mind. This will help distinguish between whether you have major depression, such as in PPD, or just a harmless case of baby blues. Remember that there is nothing to be ashamed about. This is a fairly common procedure, and you need to be open with your doctor because they can only help you if they know what's wrong.[56]

As part of the evaluation, your doctor will:

- Screen for depression by asking questions or getting you to fill out a questionnaire
- Get blood samples to check for an underactive thyroid condition, as it can also cause such symptoms
- Order other tests, if needed, to rule out other potential causes for your symptoms[56]

How to Deal With Postpartum Depression?

Aside from proper medical treatment, you will need to adjust your lifestyle to facilitate the recovery process. These include the following guidelines:

- Make healthy choices, like exercising, going for a walk, getting enough rest, eating healthy foods, and refraining from alcohol and other junk. Also, sleep or rest when your baby sleeps.
- Set realistic expectations. You will not get better overnight, and that's okay. Things will take some time to go back to normal; you just need to hang in there and keep pushing.
- Put yourself first. Take some time out for yourself. Get your partner or a babysitter to take care of the baby and invest some time doing things you enjoy. Reconnect with your partner. Get support from friends and family.

- Don't be alone. They say an idle mind is the devil's workshop, so avoid isolation. You won't feel better if you stay cooped up in your home. Get out and meet people to feel alive again.
- Don't be afraid to ask for help. Try and open up to your loved ones. Share how you feel and if they offer to help out with the baby, take them up on their offer every once in a while. Remember that you can only nurture your baby if you are nurtured yourself.

Still, if you have suicidal thoughts or thoughts about harming your baby, reach out to a friend or family member immediately. If they're not available, consider contacting 911 or your local emergency assistance number for help. Maybe even call a mental health professional or a suicide hotline. You can also contact a spiritual leader—basically, anybody that you are comfortable with. Remember that the sooner you get help, the sooner it will all be over. Also, if you think one of your loved ones is in such a situation, be sure to help them seek medical guidance at once.[56]

Are There Any Viable Treatments for PPD?

The treatment and recovery time may vary for specific patients depending on the severity of the condition and the exact symptoms they are experiencing. You won't need any particular treatment for baby blues since they usually go away on their own. Nevertheless, you should rest as much as possible and seek support from your social circle. Connect with new moms and loved ones. And avoid drugs and alcohol to avoid worsening the condition.[56]

For a patient with postpartum depression, the doctor might recommend psychotherapy, medication, or both. This will also depend on the symptoms and severity of the disease. By talking to a psychotherapist, you can learn to cope and respond better. Your doctor might also prescribe anti-anxiety or antidepressant pills. If you're breastfeeding, be sure to tell your doctor so that they give you medicine that won't harm your baby. For severe cases, you might even get an IV of brexanolone.[54]

Common Myths About Postpartum Depression

There is a lot of misinformation floating around about postpartum depression, but we're here to debunk those damaging myths that tend to generate stigma because PPD is normal—it's not your fault, and it's not something to be ashamed of.

It's Just the Baby Blues

Baby blues last for only a week or so, and any longer is a warning sign. If you feel severely depressed or anxious for weeks or months after birth, seek help.[55]

It Starts Right After Birth

PPD can occur at almost any point during the first year after you give birth. The onset can be different for different people, though most people start developing symptoms about 3 to 4 months after the baby is born. Nonetheless, late-onset can occur even a year after the baby's birth.[57]

It Will Go Away On Its Own

PPD will not go away on its own. It is a medical condition, and just like any other medical illness, you will need treatment to get better and avoid complications.

Only Women Get PPD

Fathers can also be affected by PPD because they also experience hormonal changes, like a drop in testosterone levels, and stress that is normal when having a baby. PPD in fathers usually appears 3 to 6 months after the baby is born.[57] Some studies show that around 10% of new fathers get PPD, and they are also likely to be depressed if their partner is experiencing PPD symptoms.[55]

It Can Be Prevented

Sure, you can take care of yourself to try and avoid PPD, but there really is no sure-shot way to prevent PPD. If you have a history of depression or specifically postpartum depression, inform your doctor beforehand so that you can work towards a safer pregnancy.[55]

You Hear Voices

PPD patients are not paranoid or manic. Although, of course, in severe cases of postpartum psychosis, patients might feel delusional or even have thoughts of harming themselves or their baby.[55]

You're a Bad Parent

Just like any other illness, PPD is not the victim's fault. You cannot control it, and it does not make you a failure or a bad parent. It also does not mean that you don't love your baby. Depression is a mental disorder that can affect your relationship with your baby, but it doesn't mean you don't love them.

Women With PPD Harm Their Babies

Women with PPD don't harm their babies. Thoughts of harming your baby only occur in cases of postpartum psychosis, which is extremely rare. In fact, a mother is more likely to harm herself rather than her baby in a depressive fit of PPD.[57]

Women With PPD Cry All the Time

Not all women with PPD experience the same symptoms. Some mothers might cry, some might put on a brave façade, and others might experience mood fluctuations.[57]

The Bottomline

Postpartum depression is as real as it gets, but it is nothing to be ashamed of. It is pretty common for new moms and even dads to experience baby blues initially after their baby is born. However, if the symptoms persist longer, then there might be a problem such as postpartum depression. PPD patients must be given due medical assistance immediately to avoid the complications or development of psychosis. Because remember, you can only take care of your baby if you take care of yourself.

Go ahead, Mama, take a breath and soften.

FOR ANY STAGE OF WOMANHOOD: YOU ARE WORTH IT

We are strong, but that does not mean that our bodies are invincible. No matter what stage of life we are currently in, we may come across several uniquely female issues—incontinence, pelvic dysfunction, even back pain. Common enough ailments with simply enough treatment. The problem is, there are often stigmas attached to these problems, and historically, we have been expected to work through them on our own. I am here to say, no more.

Incontinence: No, You Shouldn't Be Peeing When You Sneeze

How often have you had the urge to sneeze, but instead of grabbing a tissue, you rush to squeeze your legs together and say a little prayer? You may get some pitying laughs in public and other women may even give you a knowing pat on the back. This might be the reason so many of us think it is normal to experience incontinence early in life when it is anything but.

Unfortunately giving birth can weaken the muscles around the bladder and pelvis, and it can take between three to six months for your body to fully recover. Hitting the gym too early can cause significant incontinence problems, so if you notice bladder weakness during a workout, stop and switch to something less intensive. If you are experiencing or have experienced urinary incontinence and were told your pelvic floor is weak by a healthcare professional who was NOT a pelvic floor PT, you are not alone.

A huge myth in women's health is that if you are experiencing any pelvic pain, incontinence (or involuntary bladder leaking), urinary or bowel issues, or sexual dysfunction, you have a weak pelvic floor. Here's the truth: it is more common for the pelvic floor muscles to be hypertonic and/or uncoordinated than weak. Hypertonic pelvic floor muscles simply mean that the muscles are too tight at rest, they clench when they shouldn't be clenched, and they are too overly active.[58] An uncoordinated pelvic floor means that we are simply not using the muscles correctly. This distinction matters! The issue at hand is that many well-meaning healthcare professionals, mom-bloggers, personal trainers, yoga instructors, etc. are telling you to perform Kegels to "fix" your pain, leaking, bladder urgency, constipation, pelvic pain, tailbone pain, etc.

Urinary Incontinence

Urinary incontinence is a problem with sphincter and bladder control that causes uncontrolled leaking of urine. Millions of Americans, mostly women, suffer from symptoms of urinary incontinence.[59] In addition to this, urinary incontinence is a debilitating condition that results in surgery in 1 of 9 women.[60] It can have an impact both on the health and the lifestyle of a person. There are several different causes, types, and treatments of urinary incontinence.

Anatomy of the Urinary System

To understand why incontinence becomes a problem, one must understand how the system works in general. The kidneys and the bladder are a part of the urinary tract, responsible for the function of storing and passing urine. The urine is stored in the bladder, whereas, the muscles of the lower part of the abdomen hold the bladder in place. When the bladder is not full of urine, it is relaxed. The bladder sends nerve signals into your brain to let you know that the bladder is getting full. If the bladder is normal, you can hold the urine for some time and once ready, the brain sends signs to the urethral sphincter muscles and the bladder.

This causes the urethral sphincter muscles to relax and open the urethra, the bladder muscle squeezes and forces the urine out through the urethra to empty the bladder. The sphincter muscle closes again after going to the bathroom to keep the urine in the bladder. It only opens again when the brain signals to you that you have to urinate. However, with urinary incontinence, some parts of the system do not work how they should.

The first and foremost type is **stress incontinence**. This occurs when there is pressure[61] applied on the bladder due to weak urethral sphincter muscles. Furthermore, this pressure may be exerted by simple actions like coughing, laughing, or picking up a heavy object.

The second type is **urge incontinence**. This is an unexpected, sudden, and strong urge to urinate, resulting in an involuntary loss of urine accompanied by the urgency to urinate. Individuals will often urinate all night long. The bladder contractions are a result of irritation of the bladder due to an infection or a neurological disorder.

The third type is **overflow incontinence**. Under this type, an individual will suffer from continuous dripping or leaking of urine since the bladder is not empty. This happens mainly because the bladder is overdistended as a result of impaired detrusor contractility. Again, this damage occurs due to neurological diseases, like injury to the spinal cord or multiple sclerosis.

The fourth type is **functional incontinence** (toileting difficulties). It occurs due to physical or mental obstruction. For example, the individual may be unable to go to the washroom in time, like a person suffering from arthritis may not take off their pants in time to urinate.

The last type is **mixed incontinence**: an individual may be suffering from more than one of the types above of urinary incontinence. Often, stress and urge incontinence combined.

Although it may be challenging to provide accurate statistical data as to who suffers from it since it is not adequately reported and various interpretations of urinary incontinence exist, as per an estimate, almost 423 million (aged 20 or above) people across the globe suffer from this disease.[59,60] Among the nearly 13 million Americans who suffer from urinary incontinence, it spreads to 50% of the time to people in nursing facilities (older people).[62] It has been found that 52% of the older people living in their own homes suffer from this disease.[62] In addition, 11% of the patients admitted to a hospital had this condition, and at the time of discharge, 23% of them suffered from this disease.[62]

If we talk about women specifically, 24% to 45% of them have this condition. Furthermore, 7% to 37% of the women ranging from 20 to 39 suffer from UI.[63] Among the older aged women (above 60), around 9% to 39% of women suffer from UI.[63] Another factor prevalent in women is pregnancy, which increases the risk of urinary incontinence due to hormonal changes and increased weight. During childbirth, vaginal delivery can injure muscles required to control urine, resulting in a prolapsed pelvic floor. This, in turn, leads to the shift of the bladder, uterus, and rectum towards the vagina, which causes incontinence, and women suffer from it after having a child. This is why women with natural birth have a 50% higher chance of suffering from UI after childbirth than women who undergo cesarean delivery.[63]

Among older men, statistics[64] show that 11% to 34% of men suffer from UI; among them, 2% to 11% of them undergo this daily. In men, one of the biggest sources of stress urinary incontinence increases is prostate surgery. Professionals believe that this happens either because, during surgery damage may occur to urinary sphincter muscles, or the lack of physical support due to the removal of the prostate gland. Through this evidence, it can be surmised that women are two times more likely to suffer from urinary incontinence than men.

Increased body mass index is also among the many factors that increase the risk of urinary incontinence. The extra mass exerts greater pressure on the bladder and the muscles around it, weakening them, so the urine drips out when coughing or sneezing. Furthermore, tobacco usage can also increase chances of urinary incontinence. In addition, family history often plays a role for an individual developing this disease, particularly if a close family member has the condition of urge incontinence. Other diseases, like diabetes, can exacerbate the risk of UI.

Urinary incontinence can affect an individual's quality of life. Many people are ashamed to use this word or even acknowledge that they suffer from it. It has such a profound impact on one's psychiatric health it is often cited as the ground source of depression. It can mean that someone may avoid carrying out activities they like or having a good time with family. This inculcates feelings of loneliness, which only aggravate if the issue is not resolved on time. People suffering from it may often suffer from irritation on the skin and cause it to become sore. Even though people who suffer from it may not be able to ask for help, it should be known that this disease can be cured and prevented.

Prevention is key. Sometimes the smallest of actions are the most impactful, such as:

- Maintaining a healthy weight since being overweight makes your pelvic floor muscles weak; the fatty tissue exerts pressure on the bladder.
- Resolve constipation quickly because controlling your urge to defecate can weaken the pelvic floor muscles, hence it is important to consume more fiber.
- Avoid spicy foods as they irritate the bladder.
- Stay away from alcohol as it is a diuretic by nature causing more frequent visits to the washroom.
- Drink lots of water because it allows your bladder to increase its capacity.
- Remove things like caffeine or coffee from your daily routine since it irritates the bladder. It can be replaced with herbal teas.

The above recommendations are a first line of defense, but more often than not, more specific intervention is often needed. For example, hands-on physical therapy by a pelvic health specialist can help tremendously to reduce or completely eliminate symptoms of bladder leakage and urge incontinence. This is a specialized form of physical therapy that can improve or resolve symptoms of urinary urgency, frequency, and leakage, as well as pelvic pain, constipation, and difficulty emptying the bladder. Most often what we see with our patients at my clinic who struggle with bladder frequency is that there is not a true "weakness" of the pelvic floor musculature, rather there is tissue tightness and spasms that contribute to leaking symptoms.

Mental stress can lead to an increase in autonomic nervous system activity, which can cause an increase in bladder activity. Try reducing your stress by engaging in relaxing activities, doing things you enjoy, making time to decompress, or seeing a therapist.

Drinking enough fluids will keep your urine from getting too strong. If your urine is too concentrated and appears darker in color, it can irritate your bladder, leading to more frequent urination. The best fluid to consume is water and should be prioritized, whereas certain liquids, such as alcohol, caffeinated drinks, soda, and tea, should be limited, as they can potentially irritate your bladder. Aim for six to eight (eight-ounce) glasses of fluid a day from bladder-friendly drinks such as water, fresh juice, or water-based soups.

Avoiding constipation is important for maintaining strong bladder health, as straining puts extra pressure on your pelvic floor muscles (which help with bladder and bowel control) and may weaken them. To promote healthy bowel function, aim to eat plenty of high-fiber foods like fruits, veggies, and whole grains, stay hydrated, and engage in activity for at least 30 minutes a day.

Avoid holding urine in your bladder for too long, as this can weaken your bladder muscles and make a bladder infection more likely. How often should you be urinating? Ideally, every three to four hours. Also, take your time when urinating. Rushing may not allow you to fully empty your bladder, which could also make a bladder infection more likely. Urinating in a calm manner will relax the muscles around your bladder, which makes it easier to empty it fully. Many of our patients admit to us that they sometimes hold their bladder for several hours at a time because they are unable to leave their workstations. Our teachers especially report this problem and often don't drink enough throughout the day so they can hold their bladder for these incredibly long stretches.

Despite the high success rate in treating bladder symptoms with the above methods, only 1 out of 12 people affected seeks help.[65] As we've discussed above, there are several natural treatment options and lifestyle interventions that can help you recover from your issues without the use of medication, surgery, or injections. You don't have to live your life with these frustrating symptoms!

Tips to Reduce Leaking Urine66

1. Breathe

It may sound too simple, but before you run to the bathroom, stop and breathe! This is especially important for those that have urge incontinence symptoms. When your nervous system signals that you have the urge to urinate, those that have this type of incontinence typically have a fight-or-flight response in their nervous system, and possibly anxiety from embarrassment stemming from accidents or prior events of leaking. The best way to shut off this fight-or-flight response, with the intense sense of urgency, is to squeeze your pelvic floor, and then take a slow, deep breath counting to four, pausing, and then breathing out for four seconds. This calms down the fight-or-flight response, and therefore, also the urgency.[67]

2. Squeeze before you sneeze

This is for those with stress incontinence. If you feel that you're about to sneeze or cough, be sure to contract that pelvic floor. Many women have lost the natural response to contract with increased pressure and instead bulge, just as they do when they go to the bathroom, hence the cause of leaking!

3. Don't run to the bathroom

In addition to breathing once the urge hits, calmly stand up and walk to the bathroom after a few breaths, and keep those slow, deep breaths going while you walk normally. The worst thing you can do is to run to the bathroom as it increases pressure on the bladder.

4. Stop going to the bathroom "just in case"

Only use the restroom when you actually have to go, unless of course you're about to get on a plane or a very long car ride. Many people start using the restroom so much that the bladder gets "down trained," meaning that the sensation of needing the bathroom kicks on much quicker because the bladder no longer gets filled to normal capacity, so the new "full" is actually only a percentage of what the bladder can actually hold! To slowly "up train" the bladder, try to extend the time between bathroom breaks and only go when you have to.

What Does it Mean?

Are you still finding yourself confused about how to manage your urinary leaking? Many people have some sort of incontinence during their lifetime. **The problem is that most of them allow the problem to get worse before looking for a solution.** I hope this information has given you the information you need to make a decision about what to do next. If you are currently dealing with leaking urine, whether it is new or something nagging, we are more than happy to talk to you about your personal situation at Arancia.

Story from a Sister: Amber

As a child, Amber experienced bedwetting, urinary tract infections, loss of control of the bladder, and a leaking bowel with no sensation of fullness or urge. She never saw a doctor regarding these conditions until her teen years, which led to her family self-diagnosing the problem as laziness. This, of course, added up to a very unhappy childhood. At age 12 during a basketball game, she went to shoot the ball and when she landed after jumping up to complete the shot, the impact of both feet planting onto the firm court was enough to make her completely empty her bladder.

Soaking wet and standing in a puddle of urine on the basketball court was the final blow. She had to do something more. At the age of 13, she sought advice from an OBGYN who recommended the use of uterine tampons. This is upsetting to me as a pelvic health specialist on so many levels. To not recommend pelvic physical therapy from the start and rather suggest covering up the symptoms is doing a great disservice to the patient. After a few years, Autumn's bladder incontinence got a lot worse and the UTIs were out of control as she didn't want to resort to the uterine tampons.

Now in college, her social life was holding on by a thread. She felt that she was unable to have a romantic relationship due to her incontinence and was forced to center her day around making sure she knew where all the bathrooms were. Work, family life, and travel were all very stressful.

Desperate, she did her own thorough research and found out about our clinic, Arancia PT, and learned that we specialize in pelvic health. Luckily, we were only an hour away from her. She booked a complementary discovery visit with us and finally felt there was hope. I was horrified by the treatment she had received, or should I say lack of it.

She has been seen for six sessions now, about halfway through her plan of care, and is already able to self-manage her symptoms as we continue to make progress towards her long-term goal of being able to run for three miles without leaking. We are also working towards completely eliminating episodes of bladder leakage. Autumn is an inspiration. At the young age of 22, she began with us towards a better future. She has not lost hope of finding a natural and holistic solution that provides long-lasting relief from her bladder leakage and pelvic pain **without surgery.**

BOWEL HEALTH

If you ask people who they think has the most challenging job in the world, their answer is most likely a doctor, or an engineer, or a businessman. Their possible justifications could be that they have to work very hard, have sleepless nights, or deal with stress on a daily basis.

Well, if you ask the same question to our former President Obama, his most likely answer will be, "There is no tougher job than being a mom." Yes, Mama, you read it right! This sentiment was expressed during an interview with an Iowa TV station by our 44th President of the United States.

President Obama is not alone in this sentiment. You are probably familiar with a certain Oprah Winfrey. She, at present, is one of the most popular American talk show hosts. Oprah has been known to say during interviews on her own show that being a mom is one of the hardest things a person could do. I agree. Being a mom is more than a role of biology. It is a full-time job that boasts very few breaks and even fewer moments of appreciation in the world at large. If you want to talk about hard work, sleepless nights, and daily stress, look no further because, Mama, you are there.

The postpartum stage of pregnancy is always full of challenges. Because your body underwent massive changes to accommodate your little one, you may experience several issues with various essential systems as your body begins to heal and return to a close-to-pre-pregnancy state. Your bowels are no exception.

It is normal and expected that you will experience pain during bowel movements, especially if you received a tear or incision during the delivery process. The process of pooping puts a lot of stress on the parts of your anatomy affected by the trauma of birth. It is not uncommon to still be experiencing various bowel-related disorders induced by pregnancy weeks, or even years, after the main event.

Once again, normal and expected does not mean that you are destined to live with this pain or discomfort indefinitely. When it comes to your bowels, you do have options. The majority of these conditions that cause bowel issues can be resolved with simple management modalities. Today we are going to explore how your bowels actually work, the abnormalities you may be experiencing, and how to identify a problem early to prevent pain in the future.

What is a Healthy Bowel?

You have an entire body system designed for digesting food, and the bowel is one of its parts. The digestive system runs from the mouth to the esophagus and ends at the anus. In between those structures, you will find the stomach, intestine, colon, and rectum. The bowel is the lower part of the digestive system, comprising the small intestine, colon, and rectum. The colon and rectum collectively make up the large intestine. So, technically, a bowel has two parts: a smaller region known as the small intestine and the larger region that consists of the colon and the rectum. Both are hollow muscular tubes that vary in size.

If you have a healthy bowel, that means you should have at least one bowel movement daily. There should be no straining to pass stool and no blood in your stool either. A healthy bowel will not give you tummy aches, cramps, and fecal incontinence, as these are indicators that something may be wrong.[68,69]

How Does a Healthy Bowel Work?

Ok, now that we have established what a healthy bowel looks like, let's look at how a healthy bowel should work. A healthy bowel is vital for processing the food you eat so that your body can absorb water and nutrients from it. After all, they are vital to your recovery process. It also helps with the excretion of waste material as feces. Of note, the bowel has three primary functions, which are:

1. The absorption of nutrients from the digested food by the small intestine.
2. Absorbing any leftover water and minerals from the digested food, which is carried out by the colon.
3. Storage of waste material in the rectum.

If you are passing soft, well-formed poop 1-2 times a day, it is safe to assume that the bowel is working perfectly.[70] Moreover, if you are pooping easily without any pain or having to push hard, the bowel is healthy. Also, if you can wait for a short time after feeling the urge to poop, it also indicates a healthy working bowel that is possibly in optimal condition. Likewise, the texture of your stool signifies your bowel health status. Soft, easy-to-pass, light brown in color, and sausage-shaped stools are indicative of a healthy bowel.

Bowel-related Disorders

If any part of the bowel is unable to perform its function properly, different bowel-related disorders can occur like constipation, diarrhea, irritable bowel syndrome (IBS), etc. If you feel pain during pooping, if the stools are too hard and dry, or if you see blood within the feces, it might be due to some bowel-related disorder. The color of the stool also changes in such cases.

Let's dig into the details of some common postpartum bowel-related disorders so that you can quickly help identify which condition is affecting you.

Constipation

Constipation is often characterized by infrequent bowel movements and dry, hard stool. Most cases of constipation are temporary and can be managed with dietary changes. However, if the situation persists, it can become chronic, which can cause severe complications like abdominal swelling and rectal prolapse (intestine protruding out of the anus).

These are some of the signs and symptoms you should look out for if you suspect that you are constipated:

- Hard and dry stools, which are extremely difficult and painful to pass
- Pain in the bowel area during each bowel movement
- Less than three bowel movements during the week
- Random bouts of stomach pain
- Backing up of stool in the rectum indicated by traces of pasty stool in your underwear
- Blood in the stool

After giving birth, women usually avoid going to the toilet because of the pain, however, it is essential to maintain a normal bowel routine to prevent or reduce constipation. If you find out that you are constipated, we encourage you to make some dietary changes like eating more fruits and vegetables and drinking lots of water. These foods are fiber-filled and are most likely to fix the problem. But if the situation doesn't improve within a few days to a week, you should see a doctor immediately.

Diarrhea

Diarrhea is a condition characterized by loose and watery stool. You may feel the urge to go to the bathroom four to five times a day or more. Diarrhea can be both acute (short-term) and chronic (long-term). Acute diarrhea is short-term and lasts one to two days. It can be a result of consuming bacteria-infected food and water. When this is the case, quite often, more than one person within the household is affected. Chronic diarrhea is long-term and may last for a few weeks. It causes complications like IBS, ulcerative colitis, celiac disease, and more.

Here are some of the more common symptoms of diarrhea:

- Abdominal pain
- Bloating
- Cramping
- Bloody stools
- Dehydration

Diarrhea can sometimes be the start of some other very serious condition. Consequently, it is essential for you to see a doctor as early as possible. To fix the situation, doctors usually recommend drinking lots of fluid-like glucose-electrolyte solutions that have the right balance of water, sugar, and salts. Plain water may not be very beneficial and you may opt for a drink as described by your personal medical practitioner.

Irritable Bowel Syndrome (IBS)

Irritable bowel syndrome (IBS) is more of a digestive disorder causing diarrhea, constipation, abdominal pain, gas, etc. Constipation and diarrhea are two major symptoms of IBS. Additionally, vomiting and nausea are symptoms of irritable bowel syndrome. The combined impact of all these symptoms may cause you to experience severe weight loss.

Possible treatment includes dietary changes, like eating more fiber. Laxatives are sometimes prescribed in the case of severe constipation. Your family doctor may also prescribe glucose-electrolyte solutions in case of diarrhea. It is always necessary to consult a doctor before taking any over-the-counter medicines.

Fecal Incontinence

Fecal incontinence is the inability to control bowel movements. It may cause you to pass stool involuntarily in inappropriate places regularly. It is frequently associated with constipation, but some women experience fecal incontinence following surgery. Intractable fecal incontinence is defined as fecal incontinence that does not resolve with standard treatment measures.[71]

The symptoms of fecal incontinence vary according to the type of condition you have. There are two major conditions:

1. Urge fecal incontinence occurs when you have an urge to have a bowel movement that comes on so quickly that you can't make it to the toilet in time.
2. Passive fecal incontinence occurs when you frequently soil your underwear with stool without realizing it.

Common causes of fecal incontinence include diarrhea, constipation, problems with muscles or nerves. Enemas, dietary changes, and medications, like loperamide, may help with the situation. However, most women reacquire control of their bowels a few months after giving birth.

Hemorrhoids

Hemorrhoids are characterized by swollen veins in the lower rectum and anus. If a hemorrhoid has developed inside the rectum, it is called an internal hemorrhoid, and if it is under the skin around the anus and can be seen, it is called an external hemorrhoid. Common causes of the condition include strained bowel movements, chronic diarrhea or constipation, and a low fiber diet.

Symptoms of hemorrhoids include:

- Pain in the abdomen
- Anal swelling
- Itching in the anus
- Bleeding from the anus after a bowel movement

Eating high-fiber foods, drinking plenty of fluids, and having an active lifestyle can help with the situation.[72] So once your doctor permits, do some light activity, like a walk through your house, for at least fifteen minutes a day. If you notice any of these issues, consult a doctor immediately.

Tips for Keeping Your Bowel Healthy

To ensure that you keep your bowel in optimal health, make sure your diet is healthy. You should be eating foods like oats, nuts, peas, beans, fruits, and vegetables and ensure that you drink enough water daily. Remember to engage in physical activities to stay active because it promotes the movement of food matter along your digestive tract.

Do not rush or strain on the toilet. Allow yourself enough time and get comfortable to easily empty your bowel. You can try positioning, like leaning forward with a straight back, feet raised a little, and arms on the thighs. The normal anorectal angle in standing is 80-100 degrees. With the squatting position it changes 15-20 degrees as the puborectalis muscle begins to relax, enhancing defecation. I highly recommend using a Squatty Potty or a well-placed stool, as squatting allows for the anorectal angle to straighten, so less effort is required and could potentially reduce your chances of developing hemorrhoids. If you're struggling with constipation, you may also try to sit on the toilet right after breakfast. The gastrocolic reflex is most active immediately after waking. After a meal, gastrin enhances defecation. This will help the body create a natural cycle.

Keep observing your bowel habits so you can detect any possible change at its earliest! Continue being the awesome mama that you are!

GET IT GIRL! BUT WITHOUT THE PAIN: DYSPAREUNIA

L ife is full of simple pleasures…or great big ones. When sex becomes painful, it becomes a problem physically and mentally. Many of us believe that pain or discomfort during sex is to be expected at a certain point in our life. This is untrue. Sex should be pleasurable. I am here to explain exactly why your sex life shouldn't stay between the sheets.

Dyspareunia, or painful intercourse, can be because of a range of different reasons, including psychological concerns to structural problems. Many women experience painful intercourse at some point in their lives. It can be defined as recurrent or persistent genital pain that occurs either just before or during intercourse.[73] Oftentimes, pelvic floor dysfunction plays a role in this condition.

Did you know that a whopping 84% of us experience painful intercourse following the birth of our children?![74] This isn't surprising considering what our abdominal and pelvic floor muscles go through during a C-section or vaginal delivery. We need time to heal. At least

6-8+ weeks to be exact. But after our scars have healed and we are "cleared" for sex by our OBGYN or midwife, oftentimes, our bodies are still not ready for sex. Take home message, ladies: you are not "damaged" if intercourse is still painful after your 6-week check up. It will get better.

Symptoms

Symptoms of dyspareunia are:

- Throbbing pain that lasts for hours after intercourse
- Burning or aching pain
- Deep pain during thrusting
- Pain with penetration, even with putting in a tampon
- Pain only at penetration

Factors to Consider

- Medications: they may be a major culprit! Birth control, blood pressure, and allergy meds may cause vaginal dryness.
- Anxiety or depression can affect both libido and sexual arousal.
- Conditions such as IBS, past surgical history, ovarian cysts can play a role as well.
- Lack of estrogen during breastfeeding, early postpartum as well as during menopause can lead to vaginal dryness, thinning of the vaginal tissues, and decreased libido.
- History of sexual abuse or other emotionl afactors.

Physical Causes

Although the problem can affect both men and women, it is more common in women. Women with dyspareunia have pain in the labia, clitoris, and vagina. If the pain is acute and occurs because of deep penetration, it can be because of a medical treatment or medical condition, such as:

- Hysterectomy and other pelvic surgery
- Some cancer treatments
- Vaginal dryness
- Atrophic vaginitis, which is a common condition in postmenopausal women that causes thinning of the vaginal lining
- Side effects of drugs, such as tamoxifen and antihistamines
- Allergic reaction to douches, spermicides, and clothing
- Endometriosis, which is a painful condition that causes the tissue of the uterine lining to migrate and grow abnormally inside the pelvis
- Valvular vestibulitis, inflammation of the area that surrounds the vaginal opening
- Skin diseases affecting the vaginal area, for example, lichen sclerosus and lichen planus
- Sexually transmitted diseases, vaginal yeast infection, and urinary tract infections
- Trauma that often stems from a history of sexual trauma or abuse
- Cystitis or inflammation of the bladder wall because of a bladder infection
- Fibroids or non-cancerous tumors growing on the wall of the uterus
- Irritable bowel syndrome (IBS), which is a disorder of the gastrointestinal tract

- Ovarian cysts, which are cysts resulting from a buildup of fluid inside the ovary
- Pelvic inflammatory disease (PID)–PID is an inflammation of the female reproductive organs because of an infection
- Uterine prolapse or a condition in which the pelvic organs extend into the vagina

Psychological Causes

- Depression, fear, and anxiety contribute to vaginal dryness and can inhibit sexual arousal[74]
- In addition to this, stress can also trigger tightening of the pelvic floor muscles that results in pain
- Psychological trauma

Diagnosis

Dyspareunia can be diagnosed based on the presenting symptoms. Your medical and sexual history along with a physical examination will help the doctor determine the cause of pain during intercourse. A common presenting complaint of dyspareunia is pain on touching the genitals, early and deeper penetration. The doctor will assess the symptoms and ask questions about the exact location,[73,74] length, and time of the pain.

So what can be done? Check the list of side effects on your medication bottles. Talk to your primary care physician about alternative medication options. Find a mental health counselor in your area. Find a pelvic floor physical therapist who can help you find the root cause of your painful intercourse. This isn't something you have to live with forever. This doesn't have to be a taboo topic to discuss. There are healthcare professionals, like myself, who can help you on your healing journey towards great sex.

Story From a Sister: Karley's Story

Karley has been dealing with pelvic floor pain for the last 10 years. It began after a severe skiing injury where she fell in such a way that her ski was forcefully inserted upward into her vagina, causing a massive hematoma and torn tissue. Unsurprisingly, this caused extreme pain.

The hematoma grew to the size of a large softball and her doctor wanted to do emergency surgery that very night. Karley made the call to wait it out and luckily, the swelling started to subside and the extreme pain lessened. However, she was left with a persistent burning and itching sensation in her pelvic floor muscles. Aside from having pelvic floor pain, she was also diagnosed with hypermobility, a term used to describe the ability to move joints beyond the normal range of movement, which in her case, causes stability issues, chronic tightness, and pain in her joints. After the birth of her son, she noticed more extreme pelvic pain and back pain, likely due to her ligaments becoming even more lax from the hormonal changes that take place during pregnancy.

Karley tried many therapies, but none effectively helped ease the chronic pelvic pain symptoms until she began regular treatment at Arancia, where we employed internal pelvic floor work in addition to authentic myofascial release and an awful lot of core stabilization, as she still had a large diastasis recti gap and decreased core and lower body strength overall. Upon examination, every joint in her body was out of alignment. We had our work cut out for us, but I'm happy to say she was a diligent patient and did exactly what was asked of her to enhance overall stability in her body as well as address the pelvic floor restrictions.

About 15 visits into her treatment plan and her body was taking on a more neutral and balanced alignment, her core was stronger, and her pelvic pain was greatly diminished. Three weeks later, she dared to go skiing again. Karley had yet another fall, this time fracturing her rib. This threw her entire skeleton out of alignment and really shook her confidence. The good thing was, she was already prepared and knew that she would need to continue with intensive therapy for a while longer. She decided to stay with her family and continue their vacation.

One night she went to bed wearing a cozy pair of flannel pj's and woke up with a burning, painful sensation in her groin. Karley thought it was just a vivid dream, but the sensation was so intense it woke her up. She was half asleep when she went to the bathroom to check and discovered there was a beetle lodged in the inner wall of her labia. She was absolutely horrified and tried to flick it off, only getting more anxious and flustered when the beetle wasn't budging. Karley ended up having to use a pair of tweezers to finally remove the insect. It was so stuck in there, as she pried it off, pieces of her skin tore off along with the beetle.

Now, in addition to having a fractured rib from skiing into a pole, she had pelvic pain in the form of a burning sensation every time she urinated. Karley saw her OBGYN the next day in an emergency visit and the doctor cleared her of infections and gave her some medicated ointment to place on the abrasion.

Although this is extremely rare, it is important to check your pj's before putting them on for insects, especially if you're traveling and sleeping at a resort that could potentially have more insects than if you were home. The moral of the story, don't let the bed bugs bite!

UNDERSTANDING ENDOMETRIOSIS

This one is hard. It is surprisingly common while also being functionally invisible. Getting a diagnosis is half the battle, and while the war is being waged, women who suffer from it deal with intense pain. Patients who come to me with this are often hopeless because of this and feel that traditional practices have left them down. It is my hope that you never feel that way again.

Endometriosis is a unique female reproductive disorder that causes the growth of the uterine tissue to grow outside of the uterus. This sometimes causes an inflammatory reaction that creates scar tissue, resulting in chronic pain. The tissue is mostly found in the reproductive organs, such as the ovaries and fallopian tubes, but may also be found in the rectal area, bladder, and bowel.

1 in 10 women between the ages of 15 and 49 years old has endometriosis.[75] There are a staggering 176 million women worldwide suffering from it.[75] The disorder can affect women in all stages of their reproductive years and beyond, with many still suffering during menopause.

It follows you throughout your life and for those who suffer from it, relief is not as simple as taking a pill or undergoing surgery. Though we do not know why it occurs, we do know that there are some factors that may make you more at risk. You may have a better chance of exhibiting signs of endometriosis if another woman in your family, such as your mother, has it, your period started before you were 11, or you have heavy menstrual cycles that last more than the usual seven days.

Most women first experience pelvic pain, typically around their period. This differs from typical period cramps, as women with endometriosis often have much stronger cramps that often debilitate them from daily activities. Other symptoms women experience include pain with intercourse, both before or after; pain during ovulation; pain with bowel movements during menstruation; and sometimes pain with urination. Some women experience difficulties with menstruation bleeding, including excessive bleeding or bleeding in between cycles.

The excessive bleeding and pain is due to the shedding of the tissues growing outside the uterus as well as the normal menstruation. This causes irritation and inflammation, which leads to a cascade of new pain that differs from person to person. Some may notice back pain in addition to the cramping or digestive issues. Discomfort in the pelvic area is not uncommon.

Doctors diagnose endometriosis using a few methods. They start by listening to your symptoms and talking about your medical history. You'll discuss where you have the most pain and when during your cycle it happens. The doctor will also perform a pelvic exam. During this exam, he'll look for abnormalities. However, for the doctor to feel the endometriosis, the scar tissue and cysts that formed as a result must be quite large. If the doctor feels that endometriosis may be a possibility, they may order an ultrasound, MRI, or laparoscopy surgery to explore your pelvis and see what's causing the pain.

For many women, their diagnosis comes hand in hand with a

diagnosis of infertility. Approximately 25% - 50% of women experiencing infertility have endometriosis,[76] though the true number may be much higher. Oftentimes, the more obvious symptoms of endometriosis are put on the backburner until someone is attempting to get pregnant and is finding it more difficult than expected. It is then that doctors begin to look for the signs. Resulting infertility can be linked not only to blocked fallopian tubes, but also coinciding inflammation of the reproductive system.

It is not, however, impossible to get pregnant naturally. Women with stage 1 or stage 2 endometriosis may be able to get pregnant on their own. However, with stage 3 or 4, other options should be discussed with your doctor. In these cases, endometriosis blocks the fallopian tubes, which does not allow the egg that is released from the ovary to get through the fallopian tube to meet the sperm. This makes it impossible to have a fertilized egg that can attach to the uterine wall. If the egg and sperm do unite, there is a chance that the tissue will make it impossible for the egg to attach to the uterine wall. This increases the chance of an ectopic pregnancy or tubal pregnancy. Ectopic pregnancies aren't viable and may even put the mother's life at risk.

One of the only traditional treatments or diagnosis options is surgery. If you do opt to have this surgery, your doctor will "score" your endometriosis based on the level of affliction. The scores are presented as stages, with stage 1 being the least invasive and stage 4 the worst. Typically, women with stage 4 endometriosis have the hardest time becoming pregnant and often need infertility treatment in order to conceive.

Endometriosis is known as a reproductive disorder, but it often creates GI distress, too. Many women experience painful bowel movements as well as constipation, diarrhea, bloating, gassiness, nausea, and vomiting. This is because lesions are often found in the bowel, outside the intestines, and in the rectum. This may cause issues with bowel movements during menstruation, and even afterward. Women often experience difficulty going to the bathroom and when they do, the pain is so excruciating that it feels like razor blades are ripping through the intestines and bowel.

As you can imagine, many women experience a decreased quality of life because of the complications of endometriosis. On average, women with endometriosis lose about 38% of their work productivity because of the pain and the GI distress it causes.[77] Now, this does not necessarily mean that these women are missing work. On the contrary, many women report reduced effectiveness at work rather than actual time missed. Working through the pain and discomfort means that though they are physically at work, they are seeing a huge decrease in their personal and professional development that will remain a factor in their lives long after the pain has resolved.

Women also experience difficulties with regular activities at home, including cooking, cleaning, errands, and taking care of children. Most women complain of physical ailments rather than mental health issues because of the decreased quality of life they experience while suffering from endometriosis. This does not mean that they are not affected though; it simply means that they identify the physical aspect as the most debilitating aspect, the emotional and mental consequences may be a long-time coming.

Endometriosis is tricky. As of today, there is no cure for endometriosis; there are only known ways of minimizing the pain enough to allow sufferers to lead a somewhat normal life. There are two plans of attack when traditional doctors are looking to treat someone with endometriosis: hormonal and surgical.

Since endometriosis is directly related to the rising and falling of your hormones, some doctors may suggest hormone therapy as the first resort. This may include birth control pills to limit the hormones that cause the endometriosis growths; Gonadotropin-releasing hormone

(Gn-RH) agonists and antagonists that help lower estrogen levels and prevent menstruation; or Progestin therapy, which also stops your menstruation, which helps decrease the risk of endometrial growths. These medications do carry some risk of side effects that should be considered as well.

In other cases, especially if you plan to get pregnant, your doctor may suggest surgery to remove the endometrial growths throughout your pelvis and reproductive organs. The goal is to keep the uterus and ovaries intact so they are healthy enough to support a pregnancy while extracting the invasive tissue. Though this option may seem enticing to someone who has dealt with endometriosis pain most of their life, it does come with a price. The tissue removed will typically grow back in time.

In very extreme cases, a hysterectomy and/or ovary removal is necessary. This isn't a widely used practice since it immediately puts you into menopause and it doesn't help the endometrial growths that are already present in areas other than the uterus or ovaries. It does help with the heavy bleeding, though, which for some can be a lifesaver. In the same breath, it is important to remember that undergoing a hysterectomy comes with its own complications, especially if you're still young.

Endometriosis is often misdiagnosed. Since the build-up of tissue is not visible with current imaging technology, doctors depend on a checklist of symptoms to diagnose. It takes surgery to officially confirm the condition and if that does not happen, it is common to hear of women going without treatment for long periods of time. The condition can be confused with PCOS and other common health issues that present similar symptoms.

There is a third option.

A women's health or pelvic floor physical therapist can help. Taking advantage of physical therapy will help treat your pelvic floor muscles, help with tissue restrictions, which will help decrease or eliminate the pain you feel during sex. For example, with my pelvic health patients, we always do a thorough orthopedic exam as well as a pelvic internal and external exam. We always start with a history intake where we sit down and listen to everything you have to say. You will be asked questions about your pain, symptoms, bowel and bladder habits, diet, fluid intake, lifestyle choices, career, stress levels, pregnancy history, trauma, medications, past therapy, etc.

The next step is a thorough postural examination, as changes in your skeletal alignment can and will change the length and tension of the pelvic floor musculature. I can't speak for all clinics, but in mine, we do a standing assessment first to see how you stand against gravity, followed by sitting and lying down. Misalignment can happen due to bad postural habits, desk workers, muscle weakness and imbalances, scoliosis, and leg length differences, just to name a few.

Addressing poor postural habits can directly improve your pelvic floor dysfunction. Following the postural assessment, we do a movement analysis to find out what activities, exercises, postures or movements exacerbate your symptoms. For example, if you experience stress incontinence when you laugh, cough or sneeze, or even when you pick your child up off the floor, we will try and have you mimic that action. The goal here is to try and assess the quality of your movement and to see if there are any movement pattern impairments. If there are, we will make it a point in your plan of care to address and teach proper squatting or lifting as well as bracing techniques so you can begin to see changes in your incontinence. The next step is the orthopedic assessment where we evaluate your spine, sacroiliac joints, hip joints, rib cage as well as your breathing patterns. A pelvic floor assessment is typically performed next. It is not uncommon for the evaluation to be broken up into two separate visits given the amount of assessing that needs to be done. Pelvic floor assessments should cover both internal and external exams of the vagina and/or rectum. I typically check for trigger points and tension of the tissue. We will assess the tone, strength, and quality of your tissue and muscles. Once this step is done some patient education will be given specifically to you and your diagnosis.

Last but not least, every one of my patients receives at least a 30-minute treatment after the initial exam and assessment so you leave feeling a bit different. Treatment is different for every person and condition, but to give you an idea of the types of techniques that may take place: muscle energy techniques, myofascial release, mobilization of tight joints such as hips, coccyx, lumbar or thoracic spine, bladder release, pelvic floor muscle education with manual feedback, diaphragm release work. Contact a pelvic floor physical therapist to discuss possible treatment options to help you get back to living a better life with endometriosis.

If you think you have endometriosis, I implore you to see your doctor right away. While they cannot cure it, there are ways to minimize the growth and preserve your reproductive organs for if or when you're ready to get pregnant. At the same time, seeking out a pelvic health specialist physical therapist should be right up there in the beginning stages of treatment. Professionals like myself have the tools and knowledge to guide you through this condition. We work with your body to catalyze healing on the deepest level by treating the physicality of endometriosis.

Each step in your continued journey to a healthy, happy body should be in the direction of progress. By avoiding surgery, you are avoiding treating the scar tissue and lesions many years later, while continuing to fight the endometriosis. I know it can be scary when you know you are dealing with this and that it can affect something as important as fertility and living your life pain-free. But armed with knowledge and the willingness to continue your education on what is happening within, you can fight it while preserving the health that you do possess. As of today, endometriosis does not define you.

PELVIC INFLAMMATORY DISEASE

As you prepare to learn more about your body, remember that shame has no place here. You are built the way that you are built and if you require treatment, it should be provided with professionalism and empathy. Your body is a vessel for a wonderful, unique spirit and the aim is to treat it as the precious entity that it is. When we talk about disease, in any regard, receive that information with this in mind.

Pelvic inflammatory disease is an infection of the upper genital tract that most often occurs when transmitted bacteria spread from the vagina to the uterus, ovaries, and fallopian tubes.[78] It is a polymicrobial infection that affects young women who are sexually active. Pelvic inflammatory disease presents with mild signs and symptoms. Some women do not experience any signs or symptoms, and for this reason, until you have chronic pelvic pain and have trouble getting pregnant, you might not realize you have it. 10 to 15% of women experience pelvic inflammatory disease most commonly between the ages 20 and 24.[78,79]

Each year, there are one million women estimated to be affected with pelvic inflammatory disease and 75,000 women suffer with infertility because of untreated disease resulting in damage to the uterus and fallopian tubes.[78,79]

Pathophysiology

Pelvic inflammatory disease is an inflammatory and infectious disorder that affects the upper female genital tract, including the adjacent pelvic structures, fallopian tubes, and uterus. The infection and inflammatory disease may spread to the abdomen and perihepatic structures. Menstruating women who are below the age of 25 years, have multiple sex partners, do not use contraceptives, live in areas with high prevalence of sexually transmitted diseases are usually affected with pelvic inflammatory disease. Pelvic inflammatory disease initiates as an infection that ascends in the upper genital tract from the vagina to the cervix. In pelvic inflammatory disease, chlamydia trachomatis is a predominant sexually transmitted organism.[78,79]

Microorganisms that normally inhabit the vagina usually grow in small concentrations and protect the health of the vagina. These bacteria prevent infection with other bacteria. However, when the bacteria become concentrated or grow abundantly, it can cause infection. Bacteria that normally inhabit the vagina include *Gardenella vaginalis*, *Haemophilus influence*, *Streptococcus agalactiae*, cytomegalovirus, *Mycoplasma hominis*, *Ureaplasma urealyticum*, *Mycoplasma genitalium*, *Escheria coli*, *Peptostreptococcus* species, *Prevotella bivia* and other species of *Prevotella*. In some cases, the infection is polymicrobial, which involves more than one type of microbe. In this case, the main bacteria causing the infection is usually *N. gonorrhoeae* and *C. trachomatis*. The secondary cause of infection is usually bacteria found in low concentrations in the vagina.

Signs and Symptoms

- Tenderness of cervix, ovaries, and uterus
- Mass in one or both the ovaries
- Increased heart rate
- Vulvovaginal pain
- Lethargy
- Foul-smelling and increased vaginal discharge
- Irregular bleeding after sex and in case of menstrual bleeding
- Pain while urinating
- Painful sexual intercourse
- Fever
- Pain in the upper and lower abdomen

The disease can cause mild to moderate pain, but women with symptoms of severe pain usually present with:

- High fever
- Fainting
- Vomiting
- Sharp abdominal pain

The symptoms are more likely an indication of pelvic inflammatory disease after commencing sexual activity. However, the symptoms are often similar to other health conditions.[78,79] Acknowledging the mind-body connection and emotional impact of undiagnosed chronic pain can help you fully understand and be in tune with your body completely.

Story From a Sister: Emily

For my patient Emily, it was so much more than just a headache.

Emily was often jealous of family and friends who could talk about their pain in such a cavalier and uninterested way. For them, a headache represented a night of over-indulging, or an excess of pollen in the air, or dehydration—all of which had a clear cause and a simple, direct remedy. To Emily, it seemed that everyone around her had a direct understanding of their pain as well as an obvious pathway to pain prevention or healing.

For Emily, it just wasn't that easy. The headaches she had would come at unpredictable times, never tied to a direct exterior event. Visits to her doctor offered no insight aside from the seemingly lazy response of, "Drink more water, go to bed earlier, and exercise more." Worst of all, when the headaches hit, she had no idea how to make them stop. She had visited countless medical professionals, read endless books, and endured the well-meaning unsolicited advice of others who told her she just needed to relax more. No matter how hard she tried, the pain never went away and the answers never came.

This pain was not just an inconvenience, it was an excruciating mystery. Although many patients come in to see me at my clinic for a very specific reason, they are often surprised to find the true cause of their symptoms is very far away from where they are feeling pain. Oftentimes, when one has been experiencing chronic pain for quite some time, it's easy to forget when it all began, or dull out certain memories that are less than desirable to remember. Emily was evaluated for chronic neck pain, which we did find significant restrictions anteriorly in the front of her neck as well as in the scapular area due to a lot of repetitive lifting overhead.

She had been a waitress for over nine years and had to lift a tray of food on her shoulder, which often caused her to side-bend her neck to the left or right, pending on which shoulder she was carrying the food. After about four sessions in the clinic with us, Emily did experience significant relief from her neck pain, although something was pulling from all the way down to the end of her spine that I could feel along her sacrum and tailbone wrapping around to her pelvic floor muscles. Her lower back would always light up "red" during hands-on treatment. The vasomotor reaction is something that happens during authentic myofascial release and it is characterized by blood flowing to the surface of the skin with direct compression and stretching for a period of five minutes or longer. More about authentic myofascial release later!

There is no better example of the mind-body connection. Chronic pain can present anywhere on or in the body, and for those who experience this agony without any clear or direct explanation or solution, the physical pain can quickly turn into mental anguish. While studies have repeatedly shown that chronic pain of any kind can have a severe impact on the sufferer, for the individual experiencing chronic pain from an unknown origin, the emotional and psychological impact can be crippling. Those who experience chronic pain from an unknown origin, the psychological and spiritual toll can be almost as excruciating as the physical pain.

Pain, after all, is created through the electrical signals and chemicals our brain reads and psychological trauma is often paralyzing. Many chronic pain sufferers find themselves depressed, anxious, and questioning their very faith or core moral beliefs. The tragedy, of course, is that the heightened state of mental unwell can create new physical ailments—worsening the overall impact of the chronic pain. Help is out there.

Back to Emily. It is important to me as a specialist PT to deliver more than just pain relief to my patients. That's actually the easy part of the puzzle. The more challenging part is peeling away the layers of pain and restriction to get to the root/ultimate source of injury. That is how we do our best job as clinicians so we can figure out how to keep it from returning or getting worse. In other words, our brain is the epicenter of pain—reading and translating data being presented by the physical body. The body cannot experience pain without the processing of the mind, and the direct link between physical and mental pain can create. When I began to ask Emily if she had had any trauma to her pelvic region, her face became flush and she was contemplating answering at first, I could tell. I explained again that she was in a safe space, letting her know that whatever is spoken in the clinic stays in the clinic, confidential. She then started to speak and from the sound of her voice, the small hairs on my arms were already standing up. When she was just 21 years old, Emily explained that she had a terrible fall off the top bunk of her bed while in college one evening. After having several mixed drinks at a fraternity party, she woke up to get some water thinking she was on the bottom bunk, to her surprise she was at the top. She fell off the front edge onto the pole of the bed and it went up her rectum.

This became the source of constant pain for Emily and she was always afraid to speak up to her family or doctors about it for fear of judgment. She went on to share with me that she has had a history of irregular bowel movements for years after due to the tremendous pain she experienced. It was all starting to fit now. Emily remembers through sharing her story with me that her neck pain actually began after that terrible accident. She used to be a back sleeper, but because of the pain she felt along her rectum and sacral bone, she could not tolerate any pressure at all there for several months. Emily had no other choice but to sleep on her side or her stomach, more often than not it was her stomach.

Side note: stomach sleeping is the worst position for our bodies to be in due to the nature of forced rotation it puts the cervical spine in. Stomach sleeping can put pressure on nerves and cause numbness, tingling, and nerve pain. It's best to choose another sleep position if you are a stomach sleeper.

During her fifth visit, we began to treat her pelvic floor, including the rectum, internally. The more time we spent releasing her rectal and pelvic floor restrictions, the more her neck loosened up—go figure.

Tissue holds memory and emotion. Your body remembers every single thing that ever happens to it. The human body is over 70% connected tissue, also known as fascia. Fascia is made up of collagen, elastin and the ground substance, connective tissue cells containing enzymes, lymphocytes, immune cells, and various other substances. Had we not explored Emily's history and tissue response further, she would not have gotten more than temporary relief for her nagging neck pain. More importantly, she has reconnected with a part of herself that she had shut down for so long.

While quick, direct, and simple answers might not be immediately available to the chronic pain sufferer, the power to mitigate the mental impact of the condition is. Here are a few tips we can learn from Emily's story:

- Don't give up. Modern medicine is ever-evolving. Doctors misdiagnose. Professionals can miss symptoms. The reality is, you need to be an advocate for your own healing, and be willing to keep seeking support, answers, and solutions.
- Bottling your feelings has never solved any problems, and in the case of a chronic pain sufferer, it can actually make things far worse. Consider a journal, a counselor, or a designated time of day where you can sort out your feelings.
- Find your community. While it might feel like you're all alone, know that there are millions of individuals suffering just like you, and by combining resources and supporting each other, both comfort and potential answers can follow.

Chronic pain is more than physical: it is a total attack on your mental wellbeing, your brain, and your body. Understanding the mind-body connection can help bring some relief to your emotions while you continue to seek relief for your body.

MINDEST AND MANTRAS

"The positive thinker sees the invisible, feels the intangible, and achieves the impossible." – *Winston Churchill*

For me, it all begins with the mindset. Every part of the body is intertwined in a beautiful, all-encompassing embrace. This connection, when respected, has the capability to heal from the inside out. Here, I would like to share with you some mantras that have allowed me to set a mindset of empowerment and health at every stage of my life.

Are you ready? Take time every day to visualize what you want to achieve, and visualize positive things happening in your life. Positive thoughts attract other positive thoughts so stay focused on those. Take a deep breath and repeat in your mind or aloud. Put into practice any that resonate with you.

Mantras

- My body feels. My brain thinks. Feelings or emotions are a part of releasing pain and dysfunction in my body.
- All scars, no matter how small or insignificant, need treatment.
- I cannot say "yes" to everything while saying "no" to taking care of myself.
- I am finding a way, not an excuse.
- I have faith in my body and my baby.
- You are going to be the best mom you can be.
- I believe in my body.
- With each inhale and exhale, I am connected to my body and my baby.
- I breathe, I soften, I release.
- I will not obsess over things that are not within my control.
- I love and accept my changing body.
- I am ready.
- My body is capable and strong.
- I deserve all that is good.
- I choose to stop apologizing for being me.
- I am creating a beautiful life.
- I consciously release the past and live only in the present.
- I will love myself a little more today than I did yesterday. I will make progress on my goals. I will stay committed to my growth.
- I will ask and seek help when I need it.
- I can either be happy or I can be right.
- How can you increase your awareness so you can let go of what you need to let go of?
- I am so amazing that I cannot be ignored.
- I am present in the now.

- I am more than I appear to be, all the world's power & strength resides in me.
- Birth is safe for my baby and me.
- Contractions help to bring my baby to me.
- I accept the help of others.
- I am a good mother.
- I am a strong woman.
- I know how to take care of myself in pregnancy.
- I love my baby.
- I will make the right decisions for my baby.
- My pregnant body is beautiful.
- I accept my labor and birth.
- I am surrounded by those who love, support, and respect me.
- I know how to take care of my baby.
- I trust my body.
- I will advocate for my health.

Tips for a Healthy Mind

- Create regular gratitude and an accomplishment list.
- Let go of regrets.
- Focus on what you CAN do.
- Remove the word WRONG from your vocabulary!
- Do not work on getting rid of bad thoughts...just fill up your brain with so many good thoughts there's no more room for the bad!
- Ask yourself daily, what am I grateful for?
- Success is progress!
- Do not engage with toxic people.

- Always put yourself first.
- Take time to understand yourself.
- Value your time and energy.
- Invest in yourself: meditate, read, eat healthy food, move your body, spend time in nature, rest up, YOU ARE WORTHY.
- You are a wonder of nature, a creature of beauty, you can achieve all that you wish and more.
- The only way to heal is for there to be a mutual exchange and the willingness to do what needs to be done to find the source of the injury. You are your best ally.

SELF-CARE AND EXERCISES FOR PELVIC HEALTH BEFORE AND AFTER PREGNANCY

DISCLAIMER!

This information and content are not appropriate for every person and do not constitute medical advice. Please use caution and only under the supervision of a medical professional. Arancia Physical Therapy, LLC does not imply or express any warranty and shall not be held liable in the event of damages of any kind. Any application of this information constitutes agreement with the above terms and conditions of use. More information is available from www.aranciapt.com and please contact us if you have any questions about self-treatment or would like to speed your progress with one-on-one specialist care from Dr. Jess.

You may be wondering what you can do today to begin your journey to a happy, healthy body. Below you will find exercises I personally recommend to my clients for at-home use. When completed properly, you will feel stronger as a woman and as a mother.

Respiratory Diaphragm Release

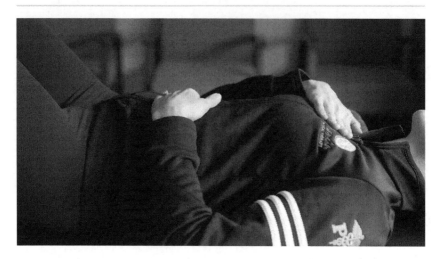

Duration: 5 minutes

Lie with the foam roller under the area of your respiratory diaphragm, just below the rib-cage.

Soften into this area for 5 minutes or until a release occurs.

Use the roller on a soft surface, such as a bed, if the pressure is too intense. You can also start propped up on your elbow and then slowly lower down as the area softens and releases.

Note: Do not do this if you have an aortic aneurysm. Reduce the pressure if you experience excessive dizziness, heart palpitations, nausea or feel you might faint.

Pelvic Floor Release

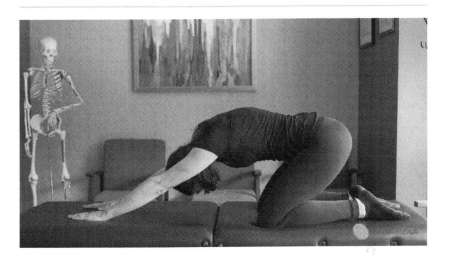

Duration: 5 minutes

Begin on hands and knees, with knees wide apart and feet close together.

Move hips back as though sitting on your heels, keeping the tailbone up. You may feel a stretch at the pelvis, hips, or back.

Gently lift the tailbone and lengthen through the inner thighs. Soften through the hips and pelvis for 5 minutes to allow several releases to occur.

Prolapse Decompression Stretches

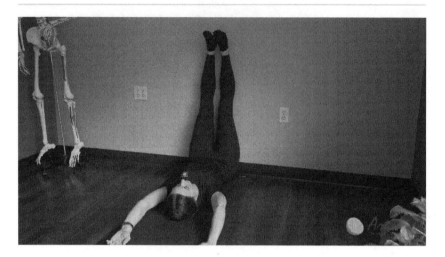

Duration: 5 minutes

Lie on the floor with your legs up against a wall.

Place your hips a comfortable distance away to allow for a gentle stretch in your legs. Keep your upper body relaxed. You may use a pillow if needed.

Lengthen through your legs and hold the stretch for 5 minutes to allow for releases to occur.

You may feel the stretch at the feet, legs, hips, pelvis, back, and even the neck.

Allow your legs to move in response to the stretch if it feels appropriate.

Note: Point toes toward the ceiling to stretch the front of the legs or press heels towards the ceiling to stretch the back of the legs. Turn toes in to stretch the outsideof the legs. Turn toes out to stretch the inside of the legs.

Allow legs to move apart to open through the inner thighs.

> *If you feel strain with your legs straight, you may need to bend your knees and let your knees relax out to the sides.

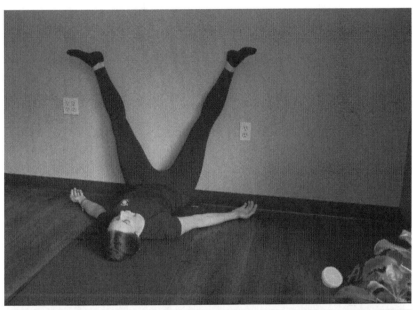

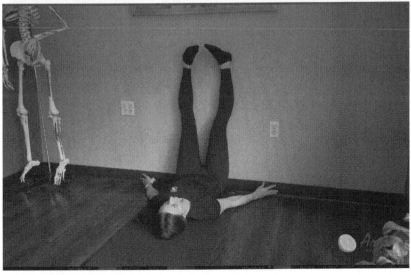

Pelvic Floor Release

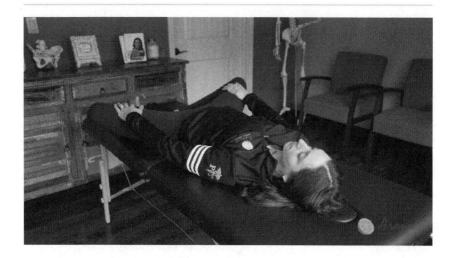

Duration: 5 minutes

Lie on your back. Bend your knees and place your feet side-by-side on the floor or bed. Drop your knees out to the sides and gently push your knees away from each other to lengthen through the inner thighs.

Hold for 5 minutes to allow for a release.

> * If this stretch is too intense, you can fold pillows or towels and place them under your knees to give some support or lessen the stretch.

Lie on your back. Bend your knees and use your hands to bring them up towards your chest and out to the sides.

Gently push your knees outwards to lengthen through the inner thighs.

Hold for 5 minutes to allow for a release.

You can also use your hands to help to release and elongate the pelvic floor and inner thighs. Place your hands on the thighs close to the pelvis, sink into the muscles, then stretch outwards towards the knees while also actively elongating.

Spine Stretch

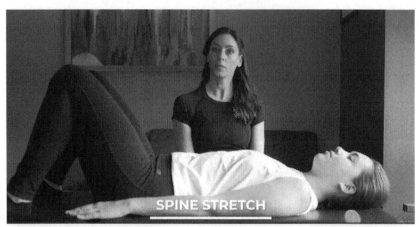

SPINE STRETCH

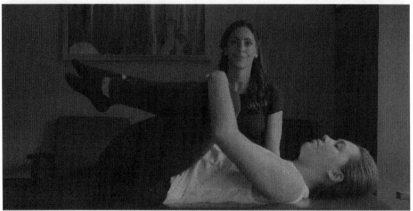

Duration: 5 minutes

Lie on your back and place the base of your skull on the top edge of the foam roller.

Allow your chin to tuck towards your chest and shoulders to relax towards the floor while lengthening through your neck and spine.

Hold for 5 minutes.

CONCLUSION

irl, you are wonderful. I say wonderful because each moment of your life, from the day you were first placed in your own mother's arms to the day that your own child was placed in yours and beyond, your body has worked in wondrous, beautiful ways. It is complicated but simple, purposeful but chaotic. It is *you*.

The world tells us that there is an empirical value assigned to each stage of life that we travel through and we are often left to navigate it alone. As children, we must learn to love who we are becoming. As teens, we must learn to be content with who we are. As young women, we must find joy in what this body can do. As mothers, we must learn to share that joy. Growing and changing are where we take charge of our own value and find empowerment in truly understanding our bodies.

If you are in the pre-pregnancy stage, sit down and prepare. Find your physical therapist, build your birth plan, gather your support team. Ready your mind and body because the plans you have will take you for the ride of your life. You are at the precipice and that rush of excitement you feel is only the beginning.

If you are pregnant, welcome! Whether you are 1 month in or 8 months along, get yourself a pelvic health assessment. Find out where you are and what you can do at this very moment to bring peace to this beautiful pregnancy. Find your mantra or repeat after me, "I embrace the messiness of life as a new mom. I let go of the need to control every aspect of my day. I practice patience with myself because the best that I can do is good enough. I am grateful for this season of my life." You have a voice, use it when you speak to yourself as well as when you find yourself at your doctor's appointments. Become an advocate for yourself now.

If you are part of the postpartum club, never lose sight of what you have done. You are a miracle and you have birthed a miracle. You are about to be told you are ready to rejoin the world and will be encouraged never to miss a step. Do it—but at your own pace. This is your life, your body, and your child.

I write *Postpartum is Forever* with a smile on my face. It has been stigmatized in so many ways and we have been taught to quickly move past it. We know this is not true. Through the pages in this book, I hope you have found knowledge and confirmation of your intuition, that this is not merely a quick blip on the map, but instead a life-long honor. There is strength in postpartum and motherhood. My friend, you are strong and wonderful.

You have joined a sisterhood of hope. In you, I celebrate this stage of your life and I encourage you in your next. I am proud of you. No matter where life will lead you or what your body may endure, you are worthy of care and health. Take care, Mama, you have so much more to accomplish.

Before you do, take a moment, breathe, and soften.

ABOUT ARANCIA PT

Over the course of this book, I mentioned my clinic, Arancia PT, several times. In a way, it is my first baby. I poured my heart, soul, and passion into this clinic for many years and at the end of the day, it is where I believe I can best help patients find healing. If you are in the area, please give us a call and see how my team at Arancia PT can continue the work we have started with this book.

Arancia specializes in pelvic health and chronic pain physical therapy practice that helps clients get back to enjoying their life again. Our clients come to us because they want more than a quick fix, and more than just pain relief. They are looking at the bigger picture. They want to live a happy, fulfilling life. They find it with us.

Arancia is the only holistic practice to create customized therapy plans for each client that addresses the 3 phases to lasting physical transformation: pain relief, strength, and mobility, and long-term strategy. We approach physical therapy in this way because we can relate to the experiences our patients are having. We understand what it feels like when nothing you've tried works. We, too, have had the ugly realization that traditional therapy and medicine offer no lasting results. We speak with experience and compassion so our clients know they're seen, heard, and understood—just like we wish we had when we were hurting.

Our team treats every client thoughtfully. We impart our expertise with clarity, encouragement, and warmth. We want to educate people without patronizing or confusing them. Every word we say informs and encourages. We want to put the joy back into your life.

This is about helping you get to your outcome, whether it's gardening or picking up your grandkid or maybe even just taking a bath without pain. Everybody is different, but it's your transformation that we're here to help you create. What I want my patients to really understand is what's going on in their bodies. I love seeing people go through their own journey and understand their own roadblocks. You're going to learn how to listen to your body, follow what you feel, and become your own self-care expert. You're going to walk away knowing how to future-proof your body.

Future-proofing means I've taught you what to do and what each feeling means in your body, like what to do with those sensations. What do they mean? So they don't scare you, but instead, inform you. That way you can self-treat. You have this one house you live in; I'm going to show you how to care for it and nurture it.

You can break down our unique philosophy into 5 tenets:

1. Pain relief isn't the best thing we can do for you: pain relief is a happy byproduct, but we mainly focus on allowing you to live a mobile, independent lifestyle with confidence that your pain will not return anytime soon, without injections, painkillers, or surgeries.

2. You and one therapist…that's it! We do not have assistants, aides, or techs here at Arancia Physical Therapy. You will spend 100% of your session with a licensed physical therapist because we believe that's how healthcare should be.

3. Treatment times: you know those 30-minute sessions, in-home therapies, and out-patient therapies? The ones that, by the time they start they don't even have much time to work on things before "cooling down"? We don't like them either. That's why at Arancia PT our sessions are at least one hour long. We know that anyone living with chronic pain needs functional repetition to improve and make significant gains, and we know that 30 minutes won't help them make the progress that we know you want to see. We believe in what is best for each and every patient to help them reach their goals—not what insurance companies say they need in their plan of care.

4. We embrace a challenging but encouraging environment, without limitations. Our team loves to learn about our patients inside and out. Figuring out what motivates them best is so important. We want to learn what ways we can make therapy fun, but still help them reach their goals. We provide a supportive and encouraging environment to help them push those really hard parts that we know will help them reach new levels. We love being silly and know when to make it more focused and serious to create the balance you or your family member needs to keep getting stronger.

5. You are family. When we opened Arancia PT, we knew that we wanted it to be a place where people felt at home. Aside from the actual physical therapy part, we love hearing about what's going on in your life otherwise; so much so that it's one of the core values we practice every day. People first, clients second. We know that you need to talk about what's going on, and we are ready to listen.

Visit our website, aranciapt.com, for more information and resources. We cannot wait to see you!

BIBLIOGRAPHY

1   Unni J, Garg R, Pawar R. Bone mineral density in women above 40 years. *J Midlife Health*. 2010;1(1):19-22. doi:10.4103/0976-7800.66989.

2   Piedmont Orthopedics. Osteoporosis vs. osteopenia: know the difference. Orthoatlanta.com.   https://www.orthoatlanta.com/media/osteoporosis-vs-osteopenia-know-the-difference.

3   Nicole W. A question for women's health: chemicals in feminine hygiene products and personal lubricants. *Environ Health Perspect*. 2014;122(3):A70-A75. doi:10.1289/ehp.122-A70.

4   Pollack GH. *The Fourth Phase of Water: Beyond Solid, Liquid, and Vapor*. Seattle: Ebner and Sons; 2013.

5   Guimberteau JC. *Strolling Under the Skin: Promenades Sous La Peau; Images of Living Fascia*. DVD. ADF Video Productions; Jan. 1, 2005.

6   John Hopkins Medicine. 4 common pregnancy complications. Hopkinsmedicine.org. https://www.hopkinsmedicine.org/health/conditions-and-diseases/staying-healthy-during-pregnancy/4-common-pregnancy-complications.

7   Bozkurt M, Yumru AE, Şahin L. Pelvic floor dysfunction, and effects of pregnancy and mode of delivery on pelvic floor. *Taiwan J Obstet Gynecol*. 2014 Dec;53(4):452-8. doi: 10.1016/j.tjog.2014.08.001. PMID: 25510682.

8   Wu, JM, Vaughan, CP, Goode, PS, Redden, DT, Burgio, KL, Richter, HE, & Markland, AD. Prevalence and trends of symptomatic pelvic floor disorders in US women. *Obstetrics and gynecology*. 2014;123(1), 141.

9   Bodner-Adler, B, Kimberger, O, Laml, T, Halpern, K, Beitl, C, Umek, W, & Bodner, K. Prevalence and risk factors for pelvic floor disorders during early and late pregnancy in a cohort of Austrian women. *Archives of gynecology and obstetrics.* 2019;300(5), 1325-1330.

10   Dheresa M, Worku A, Oljira L, Mengiste B, Assefa N, Berhane Y. One in five women suffer from pelvic floor disorders in Kersa district Eastern Ethiopia: a community-based study. *BMC Womens Health.* 2018 Jun 15;18(1):95. doi: 10.1186/s12905-018-0585-1. PMID: 29902997; PMCID: PMC6003007.

11   Chen, C.C.G., Cox, J.T., Yuan, C. et al. Knowledge of pelvic floor disorders in women seeking primary care: a cross-sectional study. *BMC Fam Pract* 20, 70 (2019). https://doi.org/10.1186/s12875-019-0958-z

12   Medically reviewed by Khatri M. All about your lungs. Webmd.com. Published May 15, 2020. https://www.webmd.com/lung/ss/slideshow-lung-facts-overview.

13   Gutke A, Buissonnault J, Brook G, Stuge B. The severity and impact of pelvic girdle pain and low-back pain in pregnancy: a multinational study. *Journal of Women's Health.* 2018; 27(4): 510-517. http://doi.org/10.1089/jwh.2017.6342.

14   Katonis, P et al. "Pregnancy-related low back pain." *Hippokratia* vol. 15,3 (2011): 205-10.

15   Corso M, Grondin D, Weis CA (2016) Postpartum Low Back Pain: It is not always What You Think. *Obstet Gynecol Cases Rev.* 3:079.

16   van Benten, Pool, J., etal. "Recommendations for physical therapists on the treatment of lumbopelvic pain during pregnancy: a systematic review." *JOSPT.* July, 2014, (44) 7. Pg. 464-473.

17   Craft LL, Perna FM. The Benefits of Exercise for the Clinically Depressed. *Prim Care Companion J Clin Psychiatry.* 2004;6(3):104-111. doi:10.4088/pcc.v06n0301.

18   Lothian JA. Safe, healthy birth: what every pregnant woman needs to know. *J Perinat Educ.* 2009;18(3):48-54. doi:10.1624/105812409X461225.

19   National Institutes of Health. Roughly one quarter of u.s. women affected by pelvic floor disorders: weakened pelvic muscles may result in incontinence, discomfort, activity limitation. Sept. 17, 2008. https://www.nih.gov/news-events/news-releases/roughly-one-quarter-us-women-affected-pelvic-floor-disorders.

20   De Bellefonds C. Medically reviewed by Propst K. Diastasis recti. Whattoexpect. com. July 8, 2021. https://www.whattoexpect.com/pregnancy/pregnancy-health/diastasis-recti-and-pregnancy/.

21   Mayo Clinic Staff. Water: how much should you drink every day? Mayo Clinic. Oct. 14, 2020. mayoclinic.org/healthy-lifestyle/nutrition-and-healthy-eating/in-depth/water/art-20044256.

22   Recurrent Pregnancy Loss. uclahealth.org. https://www.uclahealth.org/obgyn/recurrent-pregnancy-loss.

23   Background Information: Miscarriage. miscarriageassociation.org/uk. https://www.miscarriageassociation.org.uk/media-queries/background-information/.

24   Mayo Clinic Staff. Miscarriage. Mayo Clinic. Oct. 16, 2021. https://www.mayoclinic.org/diseases-conditions/pregnancy-loss-miscarriage/symptoms-causes/syc-20354298#:~:text=Overview,even%20know%20about%20a%20pregnancy.

25   Young, B; Medically Reviewed by Wilson DR. What is symphysis pubis dysfunction? Healthline. Healthline.com. Updated Dec. 5, 2018. tps://www.healthline.com/health/symphisis-pubis-dysfunction#complications.

26   Howell ER. Pregnancy-related symphysis pubis dysfunction management and postpartum rehabilitation: two case reports. *J Can Chiropr Assoc.* 2012;56(2):102-111.

27   Grow by WebMD. Best exercises for symphysis pubis dysfunction. Webmd.com. https://www.webmd.com/baby/best-exercises-symphysis-pubis-dysfunction#1.

28   Ayuda, T. Medically Reviewed by Yee R. What to know about carpal tunnel in pregnancy. Baby center. Babycenter.com. Oct. 19, 2021. https://www.babycenter.com/pregnancy/your-body/carpal-tunnel-during-pregnancy_234.

29   Carpal tunnel syndrome and pregnancy. pregnancybirth&baby. Healthdirect Australia. April 15, 2021. https://www.pregnancybirthbaby.org.au/carpal-tunnel-syndrome-and-pregnancy.

30   O'Connor A. Medically Reviewed by Wu J. What to do about carpal tunnel syndrome during pregnancy. what to expect. Whattoexpect.com. Feb. 18, 2021. https://www.whattoexpect.com/pregnancy/symptoms-and-solutions/carpal-tunnel.aspx.

31   Wright C, Smith B, Wright S, Weiner M, Wright K, Rubin D. Who develops carpal tunnel syndrome during pregnancy: An analysis of obesity, gestational weight gain, and parity. *Obstet Med.* 2014;7(2):90-94. doi:10.1177/1753495X14523407.

32   Carlson, H, Colbert, A, Frydl, J, Arnall, E, Elliot, M, & Carlson, N. Current options for nonsurgical management of carpal tunnel syndrome. *International journal of clinical rheumatology.* 2010;5(1), 129–142. https://doi.org/10.2217/IJR.09.63.

33   Dundes L. The evolution of maternal birthing position. *Public Health Then & Now;* Vol. 77, No. 5. https://ajph.aphapublications.org/doi/pdf/10.2105/AJPH.77.5.636.

34   de Jonge A, Rijnders ME, van Diem MT, Scheepers PL, Lagro-Janssen AL. Are there inequalities in choice of birthing position? Sociodemographic and labour

factors associated with the supine position during the second stage of labour. *Midwifery.* 2009;25(4):439-448. doi:10.1016/j.midw.2007.07.013.

35   Felton, J. There's a really creepy reason why women mainly give birth lying down. IFLScience; IFLScience. March 2, 2018. https://www.iflscience.com/health-and-medicine/theres-a-really-creepy-reason-why-women-mainly-give-birth-lying-down-/.

36   Mselle, L.T., Eustace, L. Why do women assume a supine position when giving birth? The perceptions and experiences of postnatal mothers and nurse-midwives in Tanzania. *BMC Pregnancy Childbirth* 20, 36 (2020). https://doi.org/10.1186/s12884-020-2726-4.

37   Huang J, Zang Y, Ren LH, Li FJ, Lu H. A review and comparison of common maternal positions during the second-stage of labor. *Int J Nurs Sci.* 2019;6(4):460-467. Published 2019 Jun 20. doi:10.1016/j.ijnss.2019.06.007.

38   Gupta JK, Sood A, Hofmeyr GJ, Vogel JP. Position in the second stage of labour for women without epidural anaesthesia. *Cochrane Database Syst Rev.* 2017;5(5):CD002006. Published 2017 May 25. doi:10.1002/14651858.CD002006.pub4.

39   Royal College of Obstetricians & Gynaecologists. Perineal tears during childbirth. Rcog.org.uk. https://www.rcog.org.uk/en/patients/tears/tears-childbirth/.

40   DiFranco JT, Curl M. Healthy Birth Practice #5: Avoid Giving Birth on Your Back and Follow Your Body's Urge to Push. *J Perinat Educ.* 2014;23(4):207-210. doi:10.1891/1058-1243.23.4.207.

41   Nasir A, Korejo R, Noorani KJ. Child birth in squatting position. *J Pak Med Assoc.* 2007;57(1):19-22.

42   Gizzo S, Di Gangi S, Noventa M, Bacile V, Zambon A, Nardelli GB. Women's choice of positions during labour: return to the past or a modern way to give birth? A cohort study in Italy. *Biomed Res Int.* 2014;2014:638093. doi:10.1155/2014/638093.

43   Barasinski, C, Debost-Legrand, A, Lémery, D, & Vendittelli, F. Positions during the first stage and the passive second stage of labor: A survey of French midwives. *Midwifery,* 56, 79–85. 2018.

44   Edqvist M, Blix E, Hegaard HK, et al. Perineal injuries and birth positions among 2992 women with a low risk pregnancy who opted for a homebirth. *BMC Pregnancy Childbirth.* 2016;16(1):196. Published 2016 Jul 29. doi:10.1186/s12884-016-0990-0.

45   Berta M, Lindgren H, Christensson K, Mekonnen S, Adefris M. Effect of maternal birth positions on duration of second stage of labor: systematic review and meta-analysis. *BMC Pregnancy Childbirth.* 2019;19(1):466. Published 2019 Dec 4. doi:10.1186/s12884-019-2620-0.

46 Bordoni B, Sugumar K, Leslie SW. Anatomy, Abdomen and Pelvis, Pelvic Floor. [Updated 2021 Jul 21]. In: StatPearls [Internet]. Treasure Island (FL): StatPearls Publishing; 2022 Jan-. Available from: https://www.ncbi.nlm.nih.gov/books/NBK482200/.

47 Akhlaghi F, Sabeti Baygi Z, Miri M, Najaf Najafi M. Effect of Perineal Massage on the Rate of Episiotomy. *J Family Reprod Health*. 2019;13(3):160-166.

48 Mayo Clinic Staff. Vaginal birth after cesarean (VBAC). Mayo Clinic. Mayoclinic.org. June 9, 2020. https://www.mayoclinic.org/tests-procedures/vbac/about/pac-20395249.

49 Blandon RE, Bharucha AE, Melton LJ 3rd, et al. Incidence of pelvic floor repair after hysterectomy: A population-based cohort study. *Am J Obstet Gynecol*. 2007;197(6):664.e1-664.e6647. doi:10.1016/j.ajog.2007.08.064.

50 Ghoniem GM. Cystocele repair. Medscape. April 12. 2021. https://emedicine.medscape.com/article/1848220-overview.

51 Lines A. Tailbone pain: pregnancy and coccyx discomfort. Kidadl. kidadl.com. July 28, 2021. https://kidadl.com/articles/tailbone-pain-pregnancy-and-coccyx-discomfort.

52 Keller L. A real pain in the butt: understanding tailbone pain during pregnancy and postpartum. Elemental chiropractic. drlaurenkeller.com. May 13, 2019. https://drlaurenkeller.com/blog/2019/5/13/a-real-pain-in-the-butt-understanding-tailbone-pain-during-pregnancy-and-postpartum.

53 Office on Women's Health. Postpartum depression. Womenshealth.gov. Updated May 14, 2019. https://www.womenshealth.gov/mental-health/mental-health-conditions/postpartum-depression.

54 Bruce DF. Medically Reviewed by Smith MW. Postpartum depression. webmd.com. Updated Aug. 4, 2020. https://www.webmd.com/depression/guide/postpartum-depression.

55 Nelson, A. Medically Reviewed by Todd N. Common misconceptions about postpartum depression. Webmd.com Updated on April 19, 2021. https://www.webmd.com/depression/postpartum-depression/common-misconceptions.

56 Mayo Clinic Staff. Postpartum depression. mayoclinic.org. Published Sept. 1, 2018. https://www.mayoclinic.org/diseases-conditions/postpartum-depression/symptoms-causes/syc-20376617.

57 Village TR. Edited by Christiansen T. Medically Reviewed by Smith T. 6 myths about postpartum depression. Therecoveryvillage.com. Updated on April 19, 2021. https://www.therecoveryvillage.com/mental-health/postpartum-depression/ppd-myths/.

58 Mayo Clinic Staff. Urinary incontinence. Mayo Clinic. Mayoclinic.com. Dec 17, 2021. https://www.mayoclinic.org/diseases-conditions/urinary-incontinence/symptoms-causes/syc-20352808.

59 Nitti, VW. The prevalence of urinary incontinence. 2001. *Reviews in urology*, 3(Suppl 1), S2.

60 Wei, JT, & De Lancey, JO. Functional anatomy of the pelvic floor and lower urinary tract. *Clinical obstetrics and gynecology*. 2004;47(1), 3-17.

61 National Association for Continence. Male stress urinary incontinence. Nafc.org. https://www.nafc.org/male-stress-urinary-incontinence.

62 Macdiarmid SA. Maximizing the treatment of overactive bladder in the elderly. *Rev Urol*. 2008;10(1):6-13.

63 Mody L, Juthani-Mehta M. Urinary tract infections in older women: a clinical review. *JAMA*. 2014;311(8):844-854. doi:10.1001/jama.2014.303.

64 Shamliyan TA, Wyman JF, Ping R, Wilt TJ, Kane RL. Male urinary incontinence: prevalence, risk factors, and preventive interventions. *Rev Urol*. 2009;11(3):145-165.

65 St. Luke's Hospital. Complementary and alternative medicine: urinary incontinence. Stlukes-stl.com. Reviewed: June 15, 2016. https://www.stlukes-stl.com/health-content/medicine/33/000168.htm.

66 NHS. How to help a weak bladder. Nhs.uk. 2019. https://www.nhs.uk/conditions/urinary-incontinence/10-ways-to-stop-leaks/.

67 Leonard J. Medically Reviewed by Biggers A. Natural remedies for an overactive bladder. Medical News Today. medicalnewstoday.com 2017. https://www.medicalnewstoday.com/articles/317091.

68 Australian Government Department of Health. Bowel health. 2021. Wa.gov.au. https://www.healthywa.wa.gov.au/Articles/A_E/Bowel-health.

69 Australian Government Department of Health. What is bladder and bowel health? Aug. 2, 2019. wa.gov.au.

70 Cancer Research UK. About the bowel: coping physically. July 11, 2019. Cancerresearchuk.org. https://www.cancerresearchuk.org/about-cancer/coping/physically/bowel-problems/about-the-bowel.

71 The Women's: The Royal Women's Hospital, Victoria, Australia. Faecal incontinence. Thewomens.org.au. https://www.thewomens.org.au/health-information/continence-information/faecal-incontinence.

72 Mayo Clinic Staff. Hemorrhoids. May 12, 2021. Mayo Clinic. Mayoclinic.org. https://www.thewomens.org.au/health-information/continence-information/faecal-incontinence.

73 Seehusen DA, Baird D C, & Bode DV. Dyspareunia in women. *American family physician*. 2014;90(7), 465-470.

74 Meana M. Painful intercourse: Dyspareunia and vaginismus. *Journal of Family Psychotherapy*. 2009;20(2-3), 198-220.

75 Gargett C, Filby C, Cousins, F. 1 in 10 women are affected by endometriosis. So why does it take so long to diagnose? Aug. 10, 2020. The Conversation. Theconversation.com. https://theconversation.com/1-in-10-women-are-affecte d-by-endometriosis-so-why-does-it-take-so-long-to-diagnose-141803.

76 CureTalks Recorded Conversation with Suneeta Senapati, MD, MSCE. Managing endometriosis leading to infertility. April 10, 2019. Penn Medicine. Pennmedicine.org.   https://www.pennmedicine.org/research-at-penn/ online-research-interviews/managing-endometriosis-leading-to-infertility.

77 Della Corte L, Di Filippo C, Gabrielli O, et al. The burden of endometriosis on women's lifespan: a narrative overview on quality of life and psychosocial well-being. *Int J Environ Res Public Health*. 2020;17(13):4683. Published 2020 Jun 29. doi:10.3390/ijerph17134683.

78 Jennings LK, & Krywko DM. 2019. Pelvic Inflammatory Disease (PID).

79 Gradison M. Pelvic inflammatory disease. *American family physician*. 2012;85(8), 791-796.

Made in the USA
Middletown, DE
08 May 2022

65300971R00128